T0229102

Current Status of Metal-on-Metal Hip Resurfacing

Guest Editors

HARLAN C. AMSTUTZ, MD
JOSHUA J. JACOBS, MD
EDWARD EBRAMZADEH, PhD

ORTHOPEDIC CLINICS OF NORTH AMERICA

www.orthopedic.theclinics.com

April 2011 • Volume 42 • Number 2

SAUNDERS an imprint of ELSEVIER, Inc.

W.B. SAUNDERS COMPANY
A Division of Elsevier Inc.

1600 John F. Kennedy Blvd. • Suite 1800 • Philadelphia, PA 19103-2899.

http://www.orthopedic.theclinics.com

ORTHOPEDIC CLINICS OF NORTH AMERICA Volume 42, Number 2
April 2011 ISSN 0030-5898, ISBN-13: 978-1-4557-0479-8

Editor: Debora Dellapena

Orthopedic Clinics of North America (ISSN 0030-5898) is published quarterly by Elsevier Inc., 360 Park Avenue South, New York, NY 10010-1710. Months of issue are January, April, July, and October. Business and Editorial Offices: 1600 John F. Kennedy Blvd., Suite 1800, Philadelphia, PA 19103-2899. Customer Service Office: 3251 Riverport Lane, Maryland Heights, MO 63043. Periodicals postage paid at New York, NY and additional mailing offices. Subscription prices are $269.00 per year for (US individuals), $513.00 per year for (US institutions), $318.00 per year (Canadian individuals), $615.00 per year (Canadian institutions), $392.00 per year (international individuals), $615.00 per year (international institutions), $132.00 per year (US students), $191.00 per year (Canadian and international students). Foreign air speed delivery is included in all *Clinics* subscription prices. All prices are subject to change without notice. **POSTMASTER:** Send change of address to *Orthopedic Clinics of North America*, **Elsevier Health Sciences Division, Subscription Customer Service, 3251 Riverport Lane, Maryland Heights, MO 63043. Customer Service (orders, claims, online, change of address): Elsevier Health Sciences Division, Subscription Customer Service, 3251 Riverport Lane, Maryland Heights, MO 63043. Tel: 1-800-654-2452 (U.S. and Canada); 314-447-8871 (outside U.S. and Canada). Fax: 314-447-8029. E-mail: journalscustomerservice-usa@elsevier. com (for print support); journalsonlinesupport-usa@elsevier.com (for online support).**

Reprints. For copies of 100 or more, of articles in this publication, please contact the Commercial Reprints Department, Elsevier Inc., 360 Park Avenue South, New York, NY 10010-1710. Tel.: 212-633-3812; Fax: 212-462-1935; E-mail: reprints@elsevier. com.

Orthopedic Clinics of North America is covered in *MEDLINE/PubMed* (*Index Medicus*), *Cinahl, Excerpta Medica,* and *Cumulative Index to Nursing and Allied Health Literature.*

Printed and bound by CPI Group (UK) Ltd, Croydon, CR0 4YY

Transferred to Digital Print 2011

Contributors

GUEST EDITORS

HARLAN C. AMSTUTZ, MD
Founding Medical Director, Joint Replacement
Institute at St Vincent Medical Center,
Los Angeles, California

JOSHUA J. JACOBS, MD
Midwest Orthopaedics, Rush-St Lukes
Presbyterian, Chicago, Illinois

EDWARD EBRAMZADEH, PhD
Director, Implant Biomechanics, J. Vernon
Luck, Sr. Orthopaedic Research Center;
Los Angeles Orthopaedic Hospital,
University of California, Los Angeles,
Los Angeles, California

AUTHORS

HARLAN C. AMSTUTZ, MD
Founding Medical Director, Joint Replacement
Institute at St Vincent Medical Center,
Los Angeles, California

KATRIEN BACKERS, PhD
Research Coordinator, Department of
Orthopedic Surgery, ANCA Medical Center,
Ghent, Belgium

S.T. BALL, MD
Department of Orthopaedic Surgery,
University of California, San Diego,
San Diego, California

JON V. BARÉ, MBBS, FAorthA, FRACS
Consultant Orthopaedic Surgeon, Melbourne
Orthopaedic Group, Victoria, Australia

PAUL E. BEAULÉ, MD, FRCSC
Head of Adult Reconstruction, The Ottawa
Hospital; Associate Professor, University
of Ottawa, Ottawa, Ontario, Canada

PATRICIA A. CAMPBELL, PhD
Director, Implant Retrieval, J. Vernon Luck, Sr.
Orthopaedic Research Center; Los Angeles
Orthopaedic Hospital, University of California,
Los Angeles, Los Angeles, California

KOEN A. DE SMET, MD
Orthopedic Surgeon, ANCA Medical Center,
Ghent, Belgium

RACHID DOUBI, MD
Orthopedic Resident, ANCA Medical Center,
Ghent, Belgium

EDWARD EBRAMZADEH, PhD
Director, Implant Biomechanics, J. Vernon
Luck, Sr. Orthopaedic Research Center; Los
Angeles Orthopaedic Hospital, University of
California, Los Angeles, Los Angeles, California

ANNA FAZEKAS, MA
The Ottawa Hospital, University of Ottawa,
Ottawa, Ontario, Canada

GEORGE GRAMMATOPOULOS, MD
Orthopaedic Registrar, Nuffield Department
of Orthopaedics, Rheumatology and
Musculoskeletal Sciences, Botnar Research
Centre, University of Oxford, Oxford,
United Kingdom

THOMAS P. GROSS, MD
Surgeon, Midlands Orthopaedics, Columbia,
South Carolina

AMRE HAMDI, MD, FRCSC
The Ottawa Hospital, University of Ottawa,
Ottawa, Ontario, Canada

CATHERINE L. HAYTER, MBBS
Musculoskeletal MRI Fellow, Department
of Radiology and Imaging, Hospital for
Special Surgery, New York, New York

J.B. HULST, MD
Department of Orthopaedic Surgery,
University of California, San Diego,
San Diego, California

THOMAS J. JOYCE, PhD
Reader, School of Mechanical and Systems
Engineering, Newcastle University,
United Kingdom

JEREMY J. KALMA, BA
J. Vernon Luck, Sr. Orthopaedic Research
Center, Los Angeles Orthopaedic Hospital,
University of California, Los Angeles,
Los Angeles, California

PAUL R. KIM, MD, FRCSC
The Ottawa Hospital, University of Ottawa,
Ottawa, Ontario, Canada

DAVID J. LANGTON, MRCS
Orthopaedic Research Fellow, Joint
Replacement Unit, North Tees and Hartlepool
NHS Trust, University Hospital
of North Tees, United Kingdom; Newcastle
University, United Kingdom

MICHEL J. LE DUFF, MA
Joint Replacement Institute at St Vincent
Medical Center, Los Angeles, California

FEI LIU, PhD
Research Director, Midlands Orthopaedics,
Columbia, South Carolina

JAMES LORD, MEng
PhD Student, Newcastle University,
United Kingdom

ZHEN LU, PhD
J. Vernon Luck, Sr. Orthopaedic Research
Center, Los Angeles Orthopaedic Hospital,
University of California, Los Angeles,
Los Angeles, California

NAVJEET MANGAT, MRCS
Orthopaedic Trainee, Northern Deanery,
Newcastle, United Kingdom

ANTONI V.F. NARGOL, FRCS (Tr & Orth)
Consultant Orthopaedic Surgeon, North Tees
and Hartlepool NHS Trust, University Hospital
of North Tees, United Kingdom

HOLLIS G. POTTER, MD
Chief, Division of Magnetic Resonance
Imaging, Department of Radiology and
Imaging, Hospital for Special Surgery;
Professor of Radiology, Department
of Orthopaedic Surgery, Weill
Medical College of Cornell University,
New York, New York

SOPHIA N. SANGIORGIO, PhD
J. Vernon Luck, Sr. Orthopaedic Research
Center, Los Angeles Orthopaedic Hospital,
University of California, Los Angeles,
Los Angeles, California

THOMAS P. SCHMALZRIED, MD
Joint Replacement Institute at St Vincent
Medical Center, Los Angeles; Department
of Orthopaedic Surgery, Harbor-University of
California, Los Angeles Medical Center,
Torrance, California

**ANDREW J. SHIMMIN, MBBS,
FAorthA, FRACS**
Consultant Orthopaedic Surgeon; Director,
Melbourne Orthopaedic Group Research
Foundation, Melbourne Orthopaedic Group,
Windsor, Victoria, Australia

EDWIN P. SU, MD
Assistant Professor of Clinical Orthopedics,
Weill Medical College of Cornell University;
Orthopedic Surgeon, Department of Radiology
and Imaging, Center for Hip Pain and
Preservation, Hospital for Special Surgery,
New York, New York

KARREN M. TAKAMURA, BA
Joint Replacement Institute at St Vincent
Medical Center, Los Angeles, California

CATHERINE VAN DER STRAETEN, MD
Rheumatologist, Independent Consultant
Clinical Research, Ghent, Belgium

MAARTEN VAN ORSOUW, MD
Orthopedic Resident, ANCA Medical Center,
Ghent, Belgium

LAUREN E. WISK, BS
Department of Population Health Sciences,
School of Medicine and Public Health,
University of Wisconsin, Madison, Wisconsin

R.P. WOON, MPH
Joint Replacement Institute at St Vincent
Medical Center, Los Angeles, California

G. WU, MD
Department of Orthopaedic Surgery,
University of California, San Diego,
San Diego, California

JAMES YOON, BA
Joint Replacement Institute at St Vincent
Medical Center, Los Angeles, California

Contents

> The results of metal-on-metal hip Conserve® Plus resurfacings with up to 14 years of follow-up with and without risk factors of small component size and/or large femoral defects were compared as performed with either first- or second-generation surgical techniques. There was a 99.7% survivorship at ten years for ideal hips (large components and small defects) and a 95.3% survivorship for hips with risk factors optimized technique has measurably improved durability in patients with risk factors at the 8-year mark. The lessons learned can help offset the observed learning curve of resurfacing.

> Total hip arthroplasty (THA) results in good outcomes in function and risk for revision in older patients. However, in young, active patients, it results in an increased rate of revision and poorer outcomes. Modern metal-on-metal hip resurfacing arthroplasty (HRA) is described as an appropriate treatment of hip osteoarthritis in young, active patients. The selection of an appropriate prosthesis is critical for this patient demographic. This review compares the functional results of THA and HRA and focuses on range of motion, activity level, groin pain, patient satisfaction, restoration of normal hip anatomy, and gait.

> Resurfacing systems use press-fit, monoblock, cobalt chrome alloy acetabular sockets because of the material's ability to withstand stresses while accommodating a large femoral head. Despite the widespread use of these types of sockets for both hip resurfacing and total hip replacement, there is a paucity of literature assessing the outcomes of these cups in particular. The 10 year survivorship of the Conserve® Plus monoblock acetabular component used in this study was 98.3% with small pelvic osteolytic lesions suspected in only 2.3%. This study highlights the excellent radiographic survivorship profile of the Conserve® Plus socket.

> The evolution of patient sporting activities after hip resurfacing has not yet been studied. A scoring algorithm to quantify sporting activity was developed to compare type of activity, frequency, duration, and overall activity level in the early postoperative

resurfacing arthroplasties performed during the same period at a minimum 2-year follow-up to evaluate the initial fixation of uncemented femoral resurfacing components. The results of this study indicate that fully porous-coated femoral resurfacing components can routinely achieve reliable fixation and provide similar initial results as have been achieved with cemented fixation. Long-term results are needed to determine which type of fixation is superior for the femoral hip resurfacing component.

Failure Modes of 433 Metal-on-Metal Hip Implants: How, Why, and Wear   241

Edward Ebramzadeh, Patricia A. Campbell, Karren M. Takamura, Zhen Lu, Sophia N. Sangiorgio, Jeremy J. Kalma, Koen A. De Smet, and Harlan C. Amstutz

Metal-on-metal total hip replacements (THRs) and hip resurfacings are coming under increasing scrutiny in light of concerns that they fail because of high wear and elevated metal ions. The aim of this study was to investigate the modes of failure in a collection of 433 metal-on-metal THRs and hip resurfacings and to examine the correlations between the reasons for revision and a range of patient and implant variables considered relevant to implant wear.

A Prospective Metal Ion Study of Large-Head Metal-on-Metal Bearing: A Matched-Pair Analysis of Hip Resurfacing Versus Total Hip Replacement   251

Paul E. Beaulé, Paul R. Kim, Amre Hamdi, and Anna Fazekas

The current study measured ion release among large-head metal-on-metal hip bearings. Twenty-six patients with a modular, Profemur® TL with A-Class® big femoral head total hip replacement were matched (gender, femoral size, BMI) with a group of 26 patients with the Conserve® Plus implant hip resurfacing. Compared with HR patients, THR patients had higher median serum cobalt ion levels at 6 months (3.26 vs 1.12 µg/L, $P = .002$) 1 year (4.51 vs 1.02, $P = .002$), and 2 years (3.77 vs 1.22, $P<.001$) following surgery. No differences in chromium ions were observed. Further research is required to determine the clinical significance of elevated serum cobalt ions.

Revisions of Metal-on-Metal Hip Resurfacing: Lessons Learned and Improved Outcome   259

Koen A. De Smet, Catherine Van Der Straeten, Maarten Van Orsouw, Rachid Doubi, Katrien Backers, and George Grammatopoulos

This retrospective, consecutive case series of a single surgeon performed between 2001 and 2010 assesses the outcome following revision of metal-on-metal hip resurfacing arthroplasties (N = 113). Mean time to revision was 31 months (0–101) after primary hip resurfacing. Malpositioning of the components with associated wear-induced soft tissue fluid collections was the most frequent factor leading to failure of a hip resurfacing arthroplasty. The mid-term outcome of the revisions was satisfactory; complications occurred in 11 patients (9.7%). Six of these patients underwent a re-revision.

The Future of Hip Resurfacing   271

Thomas P. Schmalzried

With experience in metal-metal resurfacing, several opportunities to improve resurfacing technology have been identified. There is a need for better education on hip resurfacing in residency training programs. The majority of short-term complications associated with resurfacing are related to surgical technique or component position. Innovations to improve acetabular component position and *femoral-acetabular mating* are needed. Although the majority of high wear and adverse local tissue reactions (ALTR) can be prevented by proper component positioning, the variable exposure to metal particles and ions associated with metal-metal resurfacing components continues to be a concern and bearing surface technology will evolve.

Orthopedic Clinics of North America

THE CLINICS ARE NOW AVAILABLE ONLINE!

Access your subscription at:
www.theclinics.com

Foreword
Current Status of M/M Hip Resurfacing

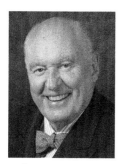

Harlan C. Amstutz, MD
Guest Editor

Few would argue that the most successful orthopedic procedure developed in the 20th century was total hip replacement (THR), and there continues to be improvement in its durability with new designs, bearing materials, and fixation techniques.

Although quite predictable and durable in older patients, young and active patients have higher revision rates,[1–7] and these rates are higher when the etiology is osteonecrosis.[8–10] Other disadvantages include the difficulty of replicating leg length and offset, maintaining proximal bone,[11–13] and the complications of dislocation,[14,15] as well as the occasional patient with annoying thigh pain.[16] In addition, revision surgery for THR generally is less satisfactory than primary THR because of diminished bone stock, hence, the consideration of resurfacing of the hip.

The concept of hip resurfacing and preserving bone has always intuitively made sense, but the first generation was plagued primarily by the high wear of the first-generation polyethylene due to the large bearing size and thin polyethylene. The new generation of resurfacings using a metal-on-metal (M/M) bearing was adopted because of low volumetric wear,[17–19] even with large diameter bearings plus the strength of the metal material that permits a thin monoblock socket, which incorporates cementless in- or on-growth surfaces for improved fixation. In addition, improved femoral bone preparation and refined cemented femoral fixation have greatly improved long-term durability. In the early procedures, the most frequent failure mode was neck fracture that is now largely avoided by proper technique.[20]

The recent data strongly support certain currently available hip resurfacing devices as being successful at 10 years in healthy males with good bone quality.[20] An expanded large study group with good bone quality and large component size is analyzed in the lead article where 99.7% of patients are surviving at 10 years. Further, survivorship has risen to 96.5% from 84% at 8 years in those challenging patients with known risk factors of small component size and cystic degeneration (see the article by Amstutz and colleagues elsewhere in this issue for further exploration of this topic).

One of the goals of resurfacing has been to enable patients to be more active with greater safety than with a THR because of the ease of revision, should it ever be necessary. Revision is generally less complex than having to revise a stem, whether it has been cemented or is cementless.[21–24] Mr Shimmin, who has extensive experience with the birmingham hip resurfacing, reviews the functionality of hip resurfacing arthroplasty (HRA), versus THR, where the advantages of HRA appear to counteract perceived disadvantages compared to THR (see the article by Shimmin and Baré in this issue for further exploration of this topic). He cited the known ceiling effect of currently used outcome studies for very active patients. This ceiling effect has been addressed by Le Duff and coworkers using a new methodology of quantifying the higher level of sporting activity allowed by many resurfacing devices (see the article by Le Duff and Amstutz elsewhere in this issue for further exploration of this topic).

Orthop Clin N Am 42 (2011) xiii–xvii
doi:10.1016/j.ocl.2011.02.002

To date, there has not been a comprehensive analysis of the results of monoblock cementless sockets used without screws in resurfacing. Hulst and coworkers report very encouraging 99.6% and 97.6% 5- and 10-year survivorship in 643 Conserve® Plus hips with follow-up of 7-14 years, with all failures occurring in small sizes (see the article by Hulst and colleagues elsewhere in this issue for further exploration of this topic).

Gross and coworkers present a preliminary experience of cementless femoral resurfacing with comparable results to a cemented version (see the article by Gross and Liu elsewhere in this issue for further exploration of this topic). A long-term analysis will be needed to determine long-term safety and efficacy.

Takamura and colleagues have performed a detailed analysis of the literature and analyzed a well-followed large series of resurfaced hips with long-term follow-up (see the article by Takamura and colleagues elsewhere in this issue for further exploration of this topic). Previous reports with short-term follow-up have demonstrated a widely varying incidence of neck narrowing with different designs and technique of implantation. Further narrowing has been reported to be a benign process that stabilized. In their study the incidence was low and, while some cases do appear to be benign and stabilize, others became associated with problems such as the occurrence of adverse local tissue reactions (ALTR) associated with high wear at longer term follow-up.[25]

In the past 3 years, ALTR, initially termed "pseudotumors," has brought a cloud over M/M implants of both HRA and especially THR, where taper fretting and corrosion may add wear in addition to the bearing wear. Many surgeons consider that the cause of tissue reactions is primarily due to allergy or hypersensitivity when in reality that is a rare occurrence. In most cases ALTR is due to increased wear from poorly positioned or designed components or both.[26–28] The recall of certain M/M resurfacing devices has brought increased visibility to this issue. Anxiety has grown among patients and surgeons despite the fact that the vast majority of M/M devices are well functioning with up to 20 years of follow-up.[29–32]

Ebramzadeh and Campbell and coworkers have updated their extensive experience reviewing failure modes of 433 retrieved devices from greater than ten thousand implanted devices from the large experience of Amstutz, De Smet, and the multicenter trials of the Conserve® Plus in the United States (see the article by Ebramzadeh and colleagues elsewhere in this issue for further exploration of this topic). In addition, numerous devices of surgeons around the world were analyzed to establish an etiology of device failure. With a complete analysis of device wear, coupled with histological analysis, the cause can be generally determined. While the exact incidence is unknown, there were a low number of cases where hypersensitivity appeared to be a factor. This also highlights the general lack of knowledge of the differences in individual response or biocompatibility. They confirmed that ALTR cases are generally associated with high wear.

There are many observations that high wear is typically associated with high serum cobalt and chromium ions. Langton reports on the relationship of design and component orientation and emphasizes the increased difficulty of using small component sizes when the socket coverage of the femoral component may be less than ideal (see the article by Langton and colleagues elsewhere in this issue for further exploration of this topic).

Further, there are reports of symptoms and signs of extremely rare cobaltism in patients with high cobalt levels in association with a M/M bearing (one of four reports in the literature and the only one with a M/M bearing).[33]

While wear issues dominate today's forums on M/M bearings, it is my view that it is not a M/M issue per se but one of device design and technique. From both the surgeons' and patients' perspective, most adverse local tissue reactions and the rare systemic toxicity are due to increased wear, which can be minimized by proper component socket design and optimized socket orientation in both the coronal and the sagittal planes. There is a special need with the smaller sizes in which the design may not provide enough socket coverage of the femoral component for lubrication to minimize wear.[28,34–39] The critical importance of these factors has not been well-understood until recently. Most surgeons believed that with a large diameter bearing, component orientation was less important because component stability was facilitated by the large ball diameter, with only rare dislocations compared to the rate of conventional THR, which is up to 7%.[14,15]

Although our understanding of resurfacing failures may not be complete, there is ample information about the various types of devices and techniques so that surgeons armed with that knowledge can minimize complications. The necessary steps to do so are detailed in this issue, in my article on incidence and prevention of complications in hip resurfacing (see the article by Amstutz and colleagues elsewhere in this issue for further exploration of this topic).

Based on our own cases, the recently identified necessity to improve socket orientation can be done with very simple attention to detail. Other surgeons have also already implemented the necessary steps to do so.

In my view, the discovery of M/M wear issues is not a true M/M issue and therefore is quite dissimilar to the problem created by first-generation THR and HRA, where ALTR was caused by particulate debris due to polyethylene wear and acrylic fragmentation. This was solved only after the main mode of failure of both THR and resurfacing—"polyethylene wear"—was identified and essentially solved 40 years after its introduction by cross-linking and sterilization in an inert environment. The introduction of cementless devices also addressed particulate-induced osteolysis by eliminating PMMA cement debris. The 10-year data demonstrating low wear of second-generation polyethylenes are promising, especially in small ball sizes but also as large as 36 mm. While there is some loss of fracture toughness and fatigue crack propagation resistance associated with these bearings, there have been very few reports of liner fractures. Polyethylene wear data with larger ball sizes up to resurfacing size and in patients with extreme activity levels similar to that observed with M/M resurfacing devices have not been published.

It has always been known that there are certain risks with each of the bearing materials used in joint replacement and this remains true today despite improved technology.

The fracture incidence of ceramics has been steadily decreasing, although the treatment of fractures, should they occur, remains challenging. The necessity of proper component orientation for ceramic-on-ceramic bearings to prevent runaway wear was identified after clinical experience and accordingly results improved and squeaking minimized.[40] Similar to the ceramic-on-ceramic bearing wear, the M/M wear issues of design and component orientation became apparent after clinical experience and there is tangible evidence that the problem is solvable. Clearly this is highly desirable since M/M is the only proven and largely successful material for resurfacing at the present time.

One of the resurfacing advantages has been the easy conversion with most reports showing morbidity and survivorship comparable to THR. However, when surgery has been delayed in association with ALTR, then revision may be more complex.

De Smet and colleagues address the important issue of revision after resurfacing failures (see the article by De Smet and colleagues elsewhere in this issue for further exploration of this topic). Their experience emphasizes the importance of revising early when failure is evident and utilizing large ball size to minimize the risk of dislocation when both components need to be revised. A maloriented socket even though well fixed should be revised. While most surgeons understand the increased difficulty of performing resurfacing compared to THR, there has been insufficient education for surgeons to gain supervised experience. In the concluding article, education, especially through resident training programs, is emphasized to produce more experienced surgeons who will use proper technique to minimize complications and to mitigate the wear issue, thereby enhancing durability.

Improved socket designs of existing devices in the future with a larger femoral head coverage by the socket should provide more flexibility for surgeons in the implantation and lessen the likelihood of increased wear despite malorientation of the socket. Instrumentation should be upgraded with some designs to aid the surgeons' ability to minimize neck fracture and facilitate the all-important positioning of the components.

Improved socket designs are already in progress to address weaknesses identified with some designs. The quality of M/M technology itself is very good when incorporated in a good design which is well positioned, but there will undoubtedly be further improvements and reduction in wear.

The choice of resurfacing as the technique of choice for most cases of arthritis is a worthy goal; however, bringing this to fruition is well in the future. It just makes sense to save the head and neck and adhere to a fundamental tenet of orthopedics espoused by our forebears—save bone.

This collection of articles has been assembled to provide a balance of information concerning the current status of hip resurfacing with a look to the future. It is my fervent desire to improve surgeon and patient education.

As Arnold Bennent said, "Any change, even a change for the better, is always accompanied by drawbacks and discomfort."

Harlan C. Amstutz, MD
Joint Replacement Institute
2200 West Third Street, Suite 400
Los Angeles, CA 90057, USA

E-mail address:
harlanamstutz@dochs.org

REFERENCES

1. Callaghan JJ, Forest EE, Sporer SM, et al. Total hip arthroplasty in the young adult. Clin Orthop 1997; 344:257–62.

2. Chandler HP, Reineck FT, Wixson RL, et al. Total hip replacement in patients younger than thirty years old. J Bone Jt Surg Am 1981;63A9:1426–34.

3. Dorr DL, Kane JT III, Conaty P. Long-term results of cemented total hip arthroplasty in patients 45 years old or younger. J Arthroplasty 1994;9(No. 5):453–6.

4. Duffy GP, Berry DJ, Rowland C, et al. Primary uncemented total hip arthroplasty in patients <40 years old: 10- to 14-year results using first-generation proximally porous-coated implants. J Arthroplasty 2001;16(Suppl 1):140–4.

5. Joshi AB, Porter ML, Trail IA, et al. Long-term results of Charnley low-friction arthroplasty in young patients. J Bone Joint Surg Br 1993;75:616–23.

6. Liang T, You M, Xing P, et al. Uncemented total hip arthroplasty in patients younger than 50 years: a 6- to 10-year follow-up study. Orthopedics 2010 Apr 16. [Epub ahead of print].

7. Georgiades G, Babis G, Hartofilakidis G. Charnley low-friction arthroplasty in young patients with osteoarthritis: outcomes at a minimum of twenty-two years. J Bone Joint Surg Am 2010;91:2846–51.

8. Beaulé P, Dorey F. Survivorship analysis of cementless total hip arthroplasty in younger patients. J Bone Joint Surg Am 2001;83-A:1590–1.

9. Min B, Song K, Bae K, et al. Second-generation cementless total hip arthroplasty in patients with osteonecrosis of the femoral head. J Arthroplasty 2008; 23:902–10.

10. Ortiguera C, Pulliam I, Cabanela M. Total hip arthroplasty for osteonecrosis. Matched-pair analysis of 188 hips with long-term follow-up. J Arthroplasty 1999;14:21–8.

11. Engh CA, Hooten JP Jr, Zettl-Schaffer KF, et al. Porous-coated total hip replacement. Clin Orthop 1994;298:89–96.

12. Dowdy PA, Rorabeck CH, Bourne RB. Uncemented total hip arthroplasty in patients 50 years of age or younger. J Arthroplasty 1997;12:853–62.

13. Rubash HE, Sinha RK, Shanbhag AS, et al. Pathogenesis of bone loss after total hip arthroplasty. Orthop Clin North Am 1998;29:173–86.

14. Callaghan JJ, Heithoff BE, Goetz DD, et al. Prevention of dislocation after hip arthroplasty: lessons from long-term follow-up. Clin Orthop 2001;393: 157–62.

15. Heithoff BE, Callaghan JJ, Goetz DD, et al. Dislocation after total hip arthroplasty: a single surgeon's experience. Orthop Clin North Am 2001;32:587–91, viii.

16. D'Antonio JA, Capello WN, Manley MT, et al. Hydroxyapatite coated implants. Total hip arthroplasty in the young patient and patients with avascular necrosis. Clin Orthop 1997;344:124–38.

17. McKellop H, Park S-H, Chiesa R, et al. In vivo wear of three types of metal on metal hip prostheses during two decades of use. Clin Orthopaed Relat Res 1996;329(Suppl):S128–40.

18. Schmalzried TP, Peters PC, Maurer BT, et al. Long-duration metal-on-metal total hip arthroplasties with low wear of the articulating surfaces. J Arthroplasty 1996;11:322–31.

19. Anissian HL, Stark A, Gustafson A, et al. Metal-on-metal bearing in hip prosthesis generates 100-fold less wear debris than metal-on-polyethylene. Acta Orthop Scand 1999;70:578–82.

20. Amstutz H, Le Duff M, Campbell P, et al. Clinical and radiographic results of metal-on-metal hip resurfacing with a minimum ten-year follow-up. J Bone Joint Surg Am 2010;92:2663–71.

21. Eswaramoorthy V, Biant L, Field R. Clinical and radiological outcome of stemmed hip replacement after revision from metal-on-metal resurfacing. J Bone Joint Surg Br 2009;91:1454–8.

22. Sandiford N, Muirhead-Allwood S, Skinner J. Revision of failed hip resurfacing to total hip arthroplasty rapidly relieves pain and improves function in the early post operative period. J Orthop Surg Res 2010;5:88.

23. Wera G, Gillespie R, Petty C, et al. Revision of hip resurfacing arthroplasty. Am J Orthop (Belle Mead NJ) 2010;39:E78–83.

24. Ball S, Le Duff M, Amstutz H. Early results of conversion of a failed femoral component in hip resurfacing arthroplasty. J Bone Joint Surg Am 2007; 89:735–41.

25. Schmalzried T. Metal-metal bearing surfaces in hip arthroplasty. Orthopedics 2009;32(9). [E-publication].

26. Langton D, Jameson S, Joyce T, et al. The effect of component size and orientation on the concentrations of metal ions after resurfacing arthroplasty of the hip. J Bone Joint Surg Br 2008;90:1143–51.

27. De Smet K, Van der Straeten C, van Orsouw M, et al. Revisions of metal-on-metal hip resurfacing: lessons learned and improved outcome. Orthop Clin North Am 2011, in press.

28. De Haan R, Pattyn C, Gill H, et al. Correlation between inclination of the acetabular component and metal ion levels in metal-on-metal hip resurfacing replacement. J Bone Joint Surg Br 2008;90:1291–7.

29. Eswaramoorthy V, Moonot P, Kalairajah Y, et al. The Metasul metal-on-metal articulation in primary total hip replacement: clinical and radiological results at ten years. J Bone Joint Surg Br 2008;90:1278–83.

30. Saito S, Ryu J, Ishii T, et al. Midterm results of Metasul metal-on-metal total hip arthroplasty. J Arthropl 2006;21:1105–10.

31. Kim S, Kyung H, Ihn J, et al. Cementless Metasul metal-on-metal total hip arthroplasty in patients less than fifty years old. J. Bone Joint Surg Am 2004;86-A:2475–81.

32. Dorr LD, Wan Z, Longjohn DB, et al. Total hip arthroplasty with use of the Metasul metal-on-metal articulation. Four to seven-year results. J Bone Joint Surg Am 2000;82:789–98.

33. Tower S. Arthroprosthetic cobaltism: neurological and cardiac manifestations in two patients with metal-on-metal arthroplasty: a case report. J Bone Joint Surg Am 2010. [Epub ahead of print].

34. De Haan R, Campbell P, Su E, et al. Revision of metal-on-metal resurfacing arthroplasty of the hip: the influence of malpositioning of the components. J Bone Joint Surg Br 2008;90:1158–63.

35. Langton D, Jameson S, Joyce T, et al. A review of 585 serum metal ion results post hip resurfacing: cup design and position is critical. American Academy of Orthopaedic Surgeons. New Orleans LA, 2010.

36. Langton D, Jameson S, Joyce T, et al. Early failure of metal-on-metal bearings in hip resurfacing and large-diameter total hip replacement: A consequence of excess wear. J Bone Joint Surg Br 2010;92:38–46.

37. Jameson S, Langton D, Nargol A. Articular surface replacement of the hip: a prospective single-surgeon series. J Bone Joint Surg Br 2010;92:28–37.

38. Langton D, Sprowson A, Mahadeva D, et al. Cup anteversion in hip resurfacing: validation of EBRA and the presentation of a simple clinical grading system. J Arthroplasty 2009;25:607–13.

39. Langton D, Sprowson A, Joyce T, et al. Blood metal ion concentrations after hip resurfacing arthroplasty: a comparative study of articular surface replacement and Birmingham Hip Resurfacing arthroplasties. J Bone Jt Surg Br 2009;91:1287–95.

40. Bader R, Steinhauser E, Zimmermann S, et al. Differences between the wear couples metal-on-polyethylene and ceramic-on-ceramic in the stability against dislocation of total hip replacement. J Mater Sci Mater Med 2004;15:711–8.

Preface
Current Status of M/M Hip Resurfacing

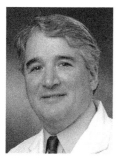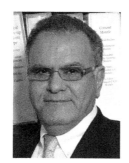

Joshua J. Jacobs, MD   Edward Ebramzadeh, PhD
Guest Editors

Over the past decade, hip resurfacing arthroplasty has made a dramatic comeback. Poor clinical results in the 1970s and 1980s resulted in many orthopedic surgeons abandoning this procedure. However, with improvements in metal-on-metal-bearing technology, new designs were introduced over the last decade to address the shortcomings in the previous generation of devices. While some reports have demonstrated excellent clinical performance of certain contemporary hip resurfacing systems, other reports have documented relatively high failure rates associated with potentially troublesome complications.

In this volume we present contributions from leaders in the area of hip resurfacing to address the current state of the science, the current controversies, and the factors associated with clinical success and clinical failure. We believe this is a timely and important addition to the orthopedic literature given the current popularity of hip resurfacing arthroplasty. As editors, we are indebted to the thoughtful and scholarly contributions of the many authors in this volume.

Joshua J. Jacobs, MD
Midwest Orthopaedics, Rush-St Lukes Presbyterian
1611 West Harrison Street, Room 300
Chicago, IL 60612, USA

Edward Ebramzadeh, PhD
Los Angeles Orthopaedic Hospital
2400 South Flower Street
Los Angeles, CA 90007, USA

E-mail addresses:
joshua.jacobs@rushortho.com (J.J. Jacobs)
EEbramzadeh@laoh.ucla.edu (E. Ebramzadeh)

doi:10.1016/j.ocl.2011.02.001
0030-5898/11/$ – see front matter

The Effect of Patient Selection and Surgical Technique on the Results of Conserve® Plus Hip Resurfacing—3.5- to 14-Year Follow-up

Harlan C. Amstutz, MD*, Karren M. Takamura, BA, Michel J. Le Duff, MA

KEYWORDS

• Hip resurfacing • Metal-on-metal • Survivorship

Metal-on-metal hip resurfacing (MMHR) is an attractive alternative to total hip replacement (THR); it provides a more anatomic and physiologic replacement, preserves more of the femoral bone, has lower dislocation rates, and has increased activity levels.[1,2] Although at short-term follow-up MMHRs have comparable results to THR[3,4] there are unique risks associated with resurfacing, such as femoral neck fracture. At short- or midterm follow-up, many studies have cited the importance of patient selection to prevent complications and optimize durability.[5–7] Early survivorship results (>5 years) range between 93% and 99.14%[8–11] and midterm results (between 5 to 10 years) between 91.5% and 95.7%.[10,12,13] The long-term performance of metal-on-metal resurfacing implants has been shown affected by component size and the presence of large defects in the femoral head.[6,14–16] Femoral size was found the best predictor of revision when all covariates were analyzed in birmingham hip resurfacings (BHR) in a study by McBryde and colleagues,[17] a result corroborated by the annual report of the Australian Orthopaedic Association National Joint Replacement Registry.[18] More recently, survivorship of hip resurfacings has been adversely affected by adverse local tissue reactions due to wear, a complication also related in part to small prosthetic size.[19,20]

The purpose of the authors' study was twofold: (1) to compare the long-term survivorship and clinical results between the hips with a femoral component size greater than 46 mm and head defects less than 1 cm (ideal hips) and those with at least one of the risk factors of femoral component size less than 46 mm and femoral head defect greater than 1 cm and (2) to assess the effects of a modified surgical technique on the survivorship of both ideal hips and hips with risk factors.

MATERIALS AND METHODS

Between 1996 and 2008, the senior surgeon (HCA) implanted 1100 Conserve® Plus MMHR (Wright Medical Technology, Arlington, Tennessee) devices in 924 patients using the cementing technique recommended for the Conserve® Plus femoral component, leaving a I-mm cement mantle.[21] The

The institution of the authors (Harlan C. Amstutz, Karren M. Takamura, Michel Le Duff) has received funding from Wright Medical Technology Inc and the St Vincent Medical Center Foundation.

Joint Replacement Institute, St Vincent Medical Center, 2200 West Third Street, Suite 400, Los Angeles, CA 90057, USA

* Corresponding author.
E-mail address: harlanamstutz@dochs.org

Orthop Clin N Am 42 (2011) 133–142
doi:10.1016/j.ocl.2010.12.005

device is manufactured as cast cobalt-chrome material, which is heat treated, solution annealed, machined, and polished. The senior surgeon made several changes to the surgical technique, which happened over time, and second-generation changes were complete by hip #300 (Table 1). Those changes were detailed in a previous study that compared the first-generation results with 6.8 years' follow-up to the second-generation results with 4.5 years of follow-up.[22] In previous reports based on a subsection of the present series, the independent effects of component size and presence of large femoral defects and body mass index (BMI) on the survivorship of the procedure were highlighted.[14,23] Although component size and femoral head defects were associated with clear cutoff marks usable for hip selection, the effect of BMI was linear rather than dichotomous[24] and did not allow suggesting value for patient selection. In addition, BMI is a variable that is associated with the patient and not the hip to be treated. Venn diagrams showing the number of hips with risk factors and the number of femoral revisions in the first and second generations show that all revisions are contained within the areas covered by small component size and large femoral defects (Figs. 1 and 2). For these reasons, the authors elected to constitute the groups studied in the present study on the basis of component size and presence of femoral defects only, although a BMI of less than 25 in combination with other risk factors substantially affects the incidence of failure. Consequently, the authors' study group was composed of 468 hips in 413 patients, selected because their femoral head size was greater than 46 mm and they presented femoral head defects smaller than 1 cm. Femoral defect size was measured from intraoperative photos, as described in a previous publication.[25] In this group, there were 404 male (97.8%)

and 9 (1.3%) female patients. The mean age of the patients was 52.1 years (range 25.4–77.5). Of these patients, 109 patients had the contralateral side resurfaced but 54 of those hips did not meet the inclusion criteria for the ideal group. All acetabular components were uncemented and all the femoral components were cemented but, in addition, the short metaphyseal stem of the femoral component was cemented in 139 out of 468 hips. In the ideal group, 205 hips were implanted with the original 5-mm shell and 263 hips with the thin 3.5-mm shell, which was introduced in October 2003 and has been used in 97% of hips since that time, enabling a larger femoral and/or a smaller socket to be inserted. The two shells were designed with identical bearing surfaces and their mechanical properties are comparable.[26]

In the hips with risk factors group, there were 632 hips in 551 patients; 323 were men (58.6%) and 228 (41.4%) were women. The mean age of the patients was 49.1 years; 302 metaphyseal stems were cemented and all acetabular components were uncemented. In this group, there were 381 hips implanted with the 5-mm shell and 251 hips with the thin 3.5-mm shell. All components were inserted using the posterior approach. Surgical details are described in a previous publication.[21] The mean duration of the follow-up period was 6.7 years (2.4–13.8) for the ideal group and 8.5 years (2.4–13.8) for the group with risk factors. The patient demographics for each group are presented in Table 2.

All follow-up examinations were performed by the senior surgeon at the authors' center or in one of the satellite clinics. These included calculation of Harris Hip Score,[27] University of California, Los Angeles (UCLA) hip scores,[28] and 12-Item Short Form Health Survey (SF-12) scores.[29] Radiographic analysis included detection of possible osteolytic lesion and measurement of

Table 1
Changes in surgical technique

	First Generation	Second Generation
Suction	No suction (first 100 hips)	Dome suction
Drilled holes	A few dome holes (0 if good bone quality)—none in the chamfered area	Increased number—chamfer holes added
Stem cementation	Stem not cemented (only in rare cases with bad bone quality)	Stem cemented in 152 regardless of cyst size
Target stem shaft angle	Anatomic (first 100 hips)	140°
Removal of cystic debris	Incomplete—curette only	Complete—high-speed burr

From Amstutz H, Le Duff M, Campbell P, et al. The effects of technique changes on aseptic loosening of the femoral component in hip resurfacing. Results of 600 Conserve Plus with a 3–9 year follow-up. J Arthroplasty 2007;22(4):481–9; with permission.

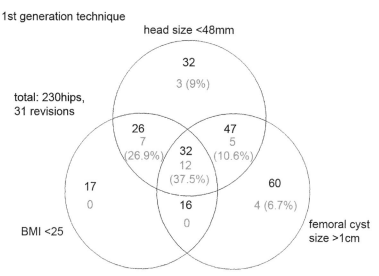

Fig. 1. Venn diagram showing the number of hips that fall into previously identified risk factor categories: low BMI (<25), large femoral cysts (>1cm), and small component size (<48mm). Overlapping areas show multiple risk factors, and the red number represents the number and percent of hips that have been undergone revision surgery for aseptic failures. This diagram shows the hips operated with the 1st generation surgical technique; hips with all three risk factors are more likely to fail with small size being the dominant factor.

the position of the components (cup abduction and anteversion) using Einzel-Bild-Roentgen Analysis (EBRA) (University of Innsbruck, Austria).[30] Using cup abduction, anteversion, and femoral head size, the contact patch to rim (CPR) distance was calculated for each hip, using a method previously described by Langton and colleagues.[31]

Two-tailed, paired, Student t tests were used to compare preoperative and last follow-up clinical scores. Two sample, equal variance t tests were used to compare last follow-up clinical scores between groups. The comparative survivorship of the ideal hips group and hips with risk factors group was assessed using standard survivorship techniques (log-rank test for comparing Kaplan-Meier survivorship curves) to account for differences in follow-up time. A P value of less than .05 was deemed significant.

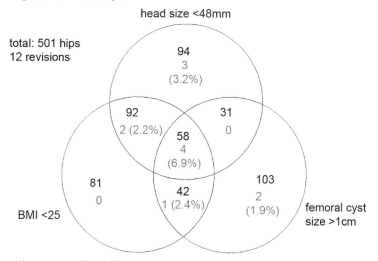

Fig. 2. Venn diagram showing number of hips with previously identified risk factors in the 2nd generation. The overlapping areas show hips with multiple risk factors, and the number in red shows the number of hips and percent that have been revised for aseptic failure. The number of revisions is insufficient to determine the predominance of a risk factor over the others.

Table 2
Patient demographics and hip reconstruction parameters compared between groups

	Ideal	Risk Factors	P Value
Male/female (%)	97.8%/1.3%	58.6%/41.4%	<.0001
BMI	28 (18.6–55.6)	26.3 (17.3–46.4)	<.0001
Age at operation (years)	52.5 (24.9–83.9)	49.1 (14.1–78.1)	<.0001
Head size (mm)	50.1	45.8	<.0001
Cup abduction	43.8° (24.8–60.0)	44.5° (16.2–71.5)	.1398
Cup anteversion	15.8° (2.0–41.8)	18.8° (2.4–55.3)	<.0001
CPR distance (mm)	16.3 (7.0–27.1)	13.5 (0.9–23.8)	<.0001
Hips with femoral defects >1 cm	0%	38.3%	<.0001

RESULTS

All mean clinical outcome scores (UCLA pain, function, walking, and activity scores) improved significantly from pre- to postoperatively as did the SF-12 mental and physical scores ($P<.0001$).

Clinical outcomes scores between ideal hips and hips with risk factors were compared and the results are in **Table 3**. There was no difference in the UCLA pain score ($P = .790$) but walking, function, and activity scores were higher in the ideal candidates ($P = .031$, $P = .006$, and $P<.0001$, respectively). The proportion of hips with UCLA activity score of 9 or 10 was greater in the ideal group (34% in ideal group vs 22% in risk factors group, $P<.0001$). The ideal hips group also had significantly higher SF-12 mental ($P = .001$) and physical scores ($P = .0055$) and Harris Hip Scores ($P = .0001$).

Radiographic Analysis

There were 4 cases of small suspected osteolytic lesions observed in the ideal hips group (0.85%) and 8 in the risk factors group (1.26%). This difference was not significant ($P = .5186$).

Ideal hips had a significantly lower average anteversion angle of 15.8° (average 2–41.8) compared with an average of 18.8° (range 2.4–55.3) for hips with risk factors ($P<.0001$). There was no significant difference in the average abduction angle between ideal and hips with risk factors. The range was wider in the hips, however, with risk factors. For ideal hips, the average acetabular abduction angle was 43.8° (24.8°–60.0°) with 12 hips (2.6%) over 55°. Hips with risk factors had an average acetabular abduction angle of 44.5° (16.2°–71.5°) with 36 hips (5.7%) over 55°.

Ideal hips had significantly larger CPR distance (median 16.3 mm, range 7.0–27.1) compared with nonideal hips (median 13.5 mm, range 0.9–23.8) ($P<.0001$).

Failures

Table 4 lists all the failures encountered in the ideal hips group and the hips with risk factors.

In the ideal hips group, there were no failures due to acetabular loosening, wear, or adverse local tissue reactions. There were two conversions to THA; 1 was revised for late sepsis at 13.1

Table 3
Clinical outcomes: ideal group versus risk factors group

UCLA Score	Ideal	Risk Factors	P Value
Pain	9.3 (3–10)	9 (2–10)	.790
Walking	9.7 (6–10)	9.6 (3–10)	.031
Function	9.6 (4–10)	9 (3–10)	.006
Activity	7.8 (3–10)	7 (2–10)	<.0001
SF-12			
Mental	54.3 (21.0–64.1)	52.6 (10.5–64.7)	<.0001
Physical	52.3 (24.1–62.4)	49.0 (17.0–67.0)	.0055
Harris hip score	95 (56–100)	92 (25–100)	.0001

Table 4 Failures		
Reason for Revision	Ideal Hips	Risk Factors Hips
Dislocation	0	1
Hematogenous sepsis	1	1
Femoral loosening	1	24
Acetabular loosening	0	4
Femoral neck fracture	0	7
Wear-related revisions	0	4
Other	0	3
Total	2	44

months postoperatively and 1 for femoral loosening 11.6 years postoperatively.

In the hips with risk factors, there were 44 revisions. Twenty-four were revised for femoral loosening, 4 for acetabular loosening, 7 for neck fracture, 4 for wear-related failure, 1 for dislocation, 1 for sepsis, and 3 for other causes (1 component size mismatch, 1 cup protrusion 3 days postoperatively, and 1 failure to achieve cup stability at surgery). There were 3 revisions for acetabular loosening in patients with thicker sockets and 1 revision in thin sockets. There were no revisions for metal hypersensitivity in either group assessed with the histologic diagnostic hallmark aseptic lymphocytic vasculitis-associated lesions).[32]

Survivorship

At both 8 years and 10 years, the Kaplan-Meier survivorship was 99.7% (95% CI, 98.1%–99.9%) for ideal candidates, with 2 revisions at 13.1 months postoperatively (sepsis) and 11.6 years (femoral loosening). For hips with risk factors, the survivorship was 91.7% (95% CI, 88.4%–94.1%) at 8 years and 84.8% (95% CI, 78.6%–89.4%) at 10 years (**Fig. 3**). This difference was significant

(log rank test, $P<.0001$). Within hips operated with the second-generation surgical technique (hip #300 and beyond), hips with risk factors had a survivorship of 95.3% (95% CI, 90.8%–97.8%) at 8 years, whereas the survivorship of ideal hips was unchanged at 99.7% at 8 years (95% CI, 97.5%–100%). This difference (**Fig. 4**) was still significant (log rank test, $P = .0338$). The survivorship improvement among hips with risk factors between first- and second-generations of surgical technique (**Fig. 5**), however, was also significant (log rank test, $P = .0231$).

DISCUSSION

Previous studies have shown that durability was better in larger components[17,18] and with cysts less than 1 cm.[23] Femoral cysts greater than 1 cm in diameter have been associated with femoral neck fractures[6,33] as well as femoral loosening.[23] There are no previous studies, however, that have looked at the combined effect of component and femoral defect size on survivorship and clinical outcomes. This study assessed the clinical outcomes of patients deemed having ideal hips based on what was found in the authors' experience and the literature to be optimal indications for metal-on-metal hip resurfacing.

The results with ideal patients were comparable to the best results reported for THR at comparable follow–up time (**Table 5**). The only aseptic failure in this group of patients happened after 11.6 years of pain-free activity in a patient whose surgery was performed with first-generation techniques and who regularly participated in ice hockey (UCLA activity of 10). Longer-term results are desirable for both types with second-generation bearing and techniques. The survivorship of ideal hips in the authors' series is 99.7% at 10 years, which

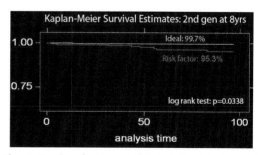

Fig. 4. Survivorship curve showing the ideal vs risk factor group with the 2nd generation surgical technique at 8 years. The ideal group still has a significantly better survivorship of 99.7% at 8 years, but the risk factor group's survivorship improves from 91.7% to 95.3% with the 2nd generation surgical technique.

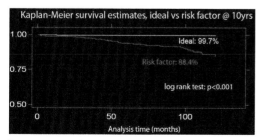

Fig. 3. Survivorship curve showing the ideal group vs the risk factor group at 10 years. Ideal candidates show significantly superior survivorship of 99.7% vs 88.4% for risk factors at 10 years.

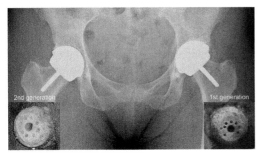

Fig. 5. X-ray of a female patient with the left hip re-surfaced with the first generation technique and the right hip resurfaced 10.5 years later with the 2nd generation technique. Both hips used the 42mm femoral component, and did not have any cysts. The left hip is almost 13 years post-op, and the right is 1.5 years post-op and both hips are doing well.

With a 10-year survivorship in ideal patients comparable to THR, the authors believe there is a clear-cut advantage of hip resurfacing because of inherent stability, consistent equal limbs, and the ease of revision it provides. Surgeons have more femoral bone stock to work with compared with THR, especially if there is extensive osteolysis in the femoral shaft. Failure of the femoral component in THR is commonly associated with some degree of bone loss and revision can be challenging.[43] Actual removal of bone at the time of implantation and bone remodeling contribute to the loss of bone stock in THR.[5] McGrath and colleagues[44] found similar clinical outcomes between primary THR and secondary THR revised from either a Conserve® Plus resurfacing or hemi-resurfacing. In the authors' series, conversion to THR was relatively simple with comparable results to primary THR.[45] The adjustment of leg length is easier with resurfacing because the bone removed from the femur is replaced by the thickness of the femoral component.

The authors' results show excellent long-term survivorship at 10 years with very low incidence of osteolysis in well-selected patients, even with 86 hips that were operated with first-generation techniques, and all of the socket components

includes both first- and second-generation surgical techniques. There was no substantial difference in survivorship between first- and second-generation techniques in the ideal hips group, which suggests that surgeons using the Conserve® Plus system who are still learning the hip resurfacing procedure can be successful with careful patient selection.

Table 5
Results of various THRs and the authors' study

Author	Year	Prosthesis	Time	Survivorship
Eswaramoorthy et al[34]	2008	Metasul MMTHR	10 y	94%
Sharma et al[35]	2007	Metasul MMTHR	12 y	95.5%
Saito et al[36]	2006	Metasul MMTHR	6.4 y	99.1%
McLaughlin et al[37]	1997	Biomet MMTHR	11y	96%
Sinha et al[38]	2004	Harris-Galante	10 y	78%
Tindall et al[39]	2007	28-mm CoCr head with full HAC-coated threaded acetabular cup (JRI Ltd) with UHMWPE insert	6 y	100%
Duffy et al[40]	2001	Harris-Galante THA	10 y	78.1%
Garcia-Cimbrelo et al[41]	2003	Zweymüller Alloclassic system THR (ceramic on polyethylene)	12 y	94.1%
Mallory et al[42]	2001	Mallory head, S-ROM series, PCA	12 y	97.5% (only femoral side survivorship given)
Ideal candidates[a]	2010	Conserve® Plus MMHR	10 y	99.7%; same as the text
Hips with risk factors[8]	2010	Conserve® Plus MMHR	10 y	84.8%
Hips with risk factors[8] (second-generation surgical technique)	2010	Conserve® Plus MMHR	8 y	95.3%

Abbreviations: CoCr, cobalt-chromium; HAC, hydroxyapatite; MMTHR, metal-on-metal total hip replacement; PCA, porous coated anatomic; UHMWPE, ultrahigh molecular weight polyethylene.
[a] Authors' current study.

were the original 5-mm thick shells. All of the components were double-heat treated and solution annealed, showing that heat treatment does not contribute to high wear and osteolysis. This result is in contrast with the claims of Daniel and colleagues,[46] who compared the 10-year survivorship of single and double heat-treated McMinn devices and concluded that double-heat treatments of metal-on-metal bearings can lead to wear-induced osteolysis and failures. Their study, however, did not measure ion levels in the patients as surrogates of wear measurement or the wear of the retrieved components, the only variables that could establish true cause and effect relationship of heat treatment on the wear of a metal-on metal prosthesis.

The complications requiring revision have occurred almost exclusively in hips with risk factors. The second-generation[24] showed significant improvements in survival rates at 8 years in hips with risk factors although a difference still exists in favor of the ideal hips. This 95.3% survival at 8 years is comparable with the results of most THR systems but can still be improved. The authors further await the longer-term results of their third-generation technique, which includes the use of a double suction and CO_2 blow-drying of the femoral head before cementation. Currently, femoral loosening and neck fractures have been virtually eliminated. There has been a gradual increase in the size of the femoral component, which provides more surface area for fixation. Further enlargement of the fixation area is obtained by meticulous bone preparation and an increase in the number of drilled holes in the chamfer and dome areas.[22] Furthermore, the authors advise using the largest head and socket size commensurate with preserving the medial wall of the acetabulum in keeping with newly established desire to increase the CPR distance to minimize wear.[31]

Except for the UCLA pain score, the authors observed higher clinical outcome scores in the ideal group compared with the risk factors group. The lower scores in the function and activity scores in the risk factors group probably reflect the authors' recommendation that patients not engage in high-impact activities; the authors' results showed that the proportion of patients who are highly active (UCLA 9 or 10) was significantly smaller in the risk factors group. In the authors' cohort, patients with ideal hips have achieved high activity levels with minimal risk (only one long-term failure in a patient with UCLA activity score of 10). Many other patients, however, regularly participate in high-impact activities, such as long-distance running, racket

sports, ballet, or martial arts; longer follow-up is necessary to assess the safety of those activities.

With a short follow-up, Garbuz and colleagues[47] and Lavigne and colleagues[48] examined the functional outcome of hip resurfacing versus large-diameter head THR in randomized, double-blind studies and found that there were no significant differences in clinical functional outcomes, including UCLA activity scores. Other studies have found that MMHR provided better clinical outcomes compared with THR, including higher activity and quality-of-life scores, but these studies did not present details of component size and bone quality in their resurfaced hips.[4,49,50] Vendittoli and colleagues[51] also examined the clinical outcomes of hip resurfacing versus 28-mm metal-on-metal THA and found that resurfacings had significantly higher Western Ontario and MacMaster Universities osteoarthritis index functional scores at 1 and 2 years postoperatively, but the differences between scores were of slight clinical relevance.

One limitation of the authors' study is the difference in BMI between the two groups. The ideal candidates had a significantly higher BMI compared with the risk factors group. In a previous publication,[24] the authors found the risk of revision lower in patients with higher BMI. Higher BMI is associated with a higher bone mineral density[52] and the patients from the ideal group may have benefited not only from fewer femoral head defect but also from better overall bone quality as a result of Wolff's law. Also, the authors found a greater CPR distance in the ideal hips group compared with the group of hips with risk factors. Smaller-size components in the hips with risk factors group accounted largely for this difference. If abduction angle of the cup was comparable between groups, however, cup anteversion was also greater in the group with risk factors, possibly an effect of most patients with developmental hip dysplasia being part of this group.

Even within a patient, one hip may be ideal for resurfacing whereas the contralateral hip may not. There were 109 bilateral patients, and 54 (50%) of the contralateral hips among those patients did not meet the criteria for ideal hips. These hips were generally the hips that became symptomatic first, more severely arthritic, and associated with cystic degeneration. This was observable both in patients undergoing simultaneous resurfacing as well as those who had a staged procedure.[53] The authors' resurfacing series is unique in the literature in that the entire series was performed with no exclusion criteria for bone quality as long as the procedure was technically feasible, as pointed out in the authors' previous publication,[14] and, therefore, the authors had a group of hips with substantial risk factors to use as controls. Prosser and colleagues[54] found that patients with osteoarthritis who were less than 55 years of age and were treated with resurfacing had a revision rate of 3% at 7 years when the femoral head size was 50 mm or greater. The authors concluded that risk factors for revisions were older patients, smaller femoral size, and patients with developmental hip dysplasia and certain implant designs. In the present series, which was exclusively performed with the Conserve® Plus design, the authors' found no association of revision with age.

The MMHR literature stresses the importance of proper patient selection.[5,7] This may be important especially for surgeons who are in the learning curve phase of hip resurfacing or those who have not carefully studied the experience of others for advantages of lessons learned to date.[10,12,55–57] When the hip is selected for good bone quality and big component size, the authors' study has shown that survivorship is greatly improved. In centers with great experience in resurfacing, the indications of the procedure[58] can safely be extended, as shown by the results of the authors' second-generation of surgical technique in patients with risk factors. These results may not be applicable for other designs, however, where there is a very thin or no cement mantle or where the femoral component coverage is inadequate. Higher than normal wear rates have become an important issue in the survivorship of metal-on-metal resurfacing, and the authors recommend using thin sockets and increasing the size of the femoral component whenever possible to increase the CPR distance and minimize wear.

REFERENCES

1. Vail T, Mont M, McGrath M, et al. Hip resurfacing: patient and treatment options. J Bone Joint Surg Am 2009;91(Suppl 5):2–4.
2. Quesada M, Marker D, Mont M. Metal-on-metal hip resurfacing: advantages and disadvantages. J Arthroplasty 2008;23(Suppl 7):69–73.
3. Mont M, Marker DR, Smith J, et al. Resurfacing is comparable to total hip arthroplasty at short-term follow-up. Clin Orthop Relat Res 2009;467(1):66–71.
4. Vail T, Mina C, Yergler J, et al. Metal-on-metal hip resurfacing compares favorably with THA at 2 years followup. Clin Orthop Relat Res 2006;453:123–31.
5. Beaulé P, Dorey F, Le Duff M, et al. Risk factors affecting outcome of metal on metal surface arthroplasty of the hip. Clin Orthop 2004;418:87–93.
6. Marker D, Seyler T, Jinnah R, et al. Femoral neck fractures after metal-on-metal total hip resurfacing:

7. Schmalzried T, Silva M, de la Rosa M, et al. Optimizing patient selection and outcomes with total hip resurfacing. Clin Orthop Relat Res 2005;441: 200–4.
8. Back D, Dalziel R, Young D, et al. Early results of primary Birmingham hip resurfacings. An independent prospective study of the first 230 hips. J Bone Joint Surg Br 2005;87(3):324–9.
9. Langton D, Jameson S, Joyce T, et al. Early failure of metal-on-metal bearings in hip resurfacing and large-diameter total hip replacement: a consequence of excess wear. J Bone Joint Surg Br 2010;92(1):38–46.
10. Amstutz H. Hip resurfacing: principles, indications, technique and results. Philadelphia: Saunders - Elsevier; 2008.
11. Witzleb W, Arnold M, Krummenauer F, et al. Birmingham hip resurfacing arthroplasty: short-term clinical and radiographic outcome. Eur J Med Res 2008; 13(1):39–46.
12. Khan M, Kuiper J, Edwards D, et al. Birmingham hip arthroplasty five to eight years of prospective multi-center results. J Arthroplasty 2009;24(7):1044–50.
13. Madhu T, Akula M, Raman R, et al. The Birmingham hip resurfacing prosthesis an independent single surgeon's experience at 7-year follow-up. J Arthroplasty 2011;26(1):1–8.
14. Amstutz H, Le Duff M. Eleven years of experience with metal-on-metal hybrid hip resurfacing: a review of 1000 conserve plus. J Arthroplasty 2008;23(6 Suppl 1): 36–43.
15. Revell M, McBryde C, Bhatnagar S, et al. Metal-on-metal hip resurfacing in osteonecrosis of the femoral head. J Bone Joint Surg Am 2006;88(Suppl 3): 98–103.
16. Amstutz H, Le Duff M, Campbell P, et al. Clinical and radiographic results of metal-on-metal hip resurfacing with a minimum ten-year follow-up. J Bone Joint Surg Am 2010;92(16):2663–71.
17. McBryde C, Theivendran K, Thomas A, et al. The influence of head size and sex on the outcome of birmingham hip resurfacing. J Bone Joint Surg Am 2010;92(1):107–12.
18. Graves S. Annual Report. Australian Orthopaedic Association—National joint replacement registry. Adelaide, 2009.
19. Glyn-Jones S, Pandit H, Kwon Y, et al. Risk factors for inflammatory pseudotumour formation following hip resurfacing. J Bone Joint Surg Br 2009;91(12): 1566–74.
20. Jameson S, Langton D, Nargol A. Articular surface replacement of the hip: a prospective single-surgeon series. J Bone Joint Surg Br 2010;92(1): 28–37.
21. Amstutz H, Beaulé P, Dorey F, et al. Metal-on-metal hybrid surface arthroplasty—surgical technique.

a prospective cohort study. J Arthroplasty 2007; 22(7 Suppl 3):66–71.

J Bone Joint Surg Am 2006;88(Suppl 1 part 2): 234–49.

22. Amstutz H, Le Duff M, Campbell P, et al. The effects of technique changes on aseptic loosening of the femoral component in hip resurfacing. Results of 600 Conserve Plus with a 3-9 year follow-up. J Arthroplasty 2007;22(4):481–9.

23. Amstutz H, Beaulé P, Dorey F, et al. Metal-on-metal hybrid surface arthroplasty: two to six year follow-up. J Bone Joint Surg Am 2004;86:28–39.

24. Le Duff M, Amstutz H, Dorey F. Metal-on-metal hip resurfacing for obese patients. J Bone Joint Surg Am 2007;89(12):2705–11.

25. Amstutz H, Ball S, Le Duff M, et al. Hip resurfacing for patients under 50 years of age. Results of 350 Conserve Plus with a 2-9 year follow-up. Clin Orthop Relat Res 2007;460:159–64.

26. Le Duff M, Wang C, Wisk L, et al. Benefits of thin-shelled acetabular components for metal-on-metal hip resurfacing arthroplasty. J Orthop Res 2010; 28(12):1665–70.

27. Harris W. Traumatic arthritis of the hip after dislocation and acetabular fractures: treatment by mold arthroplasty. An end-result study using a new method of result evaluation. J Bone Joint Surg Am 1969; 51(4):737–55.

28. Amstutz H, Thomas B, Jinnah R, et al. Treatment of primary osteoarthritis of the hip. A comparison of total joint and surface replacement arthroplasty. J Bone Joint Surg Am 1984;66(2):228–41.

29. Ware J, Kosinski M, Keller S. SF-12: how to score the SF-12 physical and mental health summary scales. 3rd edition. Lincoln (RI): Quality Metric Inc; 1998.

30. Langton D, Sprowson A, Mahadeva D, et al. Cup anteversion in hip resurfacing: validation of EBRA and the presentation of a simple clinical grading system. J Arthroplasty 2009;25(4):607–13.

31. Langton D, Sprowson A, Joyce T, et al. Blood metal ion concentrations after hip resurfacing arthroplasty: a comparative study of articular surface replacement and Birmingham hip resurfacing arthroplasties. J Bone Joint Surg Br 2009;91(10):1287–95.

32. Campbell P, Ebramzadeh E, Nelson S, et al. Histological features of pseudotumor-like tissues from metal-on-metal hips. Clin Orthop Relat Res 2010; 468(9):2321–7.

33. Amstutz H, Campbell P, Le Duff M. Fracture of the neck of the femur after surface arthroplasty of the hip. J Bone Joint Surg Am 2004;86(9):1874–7.

34. Eswaramoorthy V, Moonot P, Kalairajah Y, et al. The Metasul metal-on-metal articulation in primary total hip replacement: clinical and radiological results at ten years. J Bone and Joint Surg Br 2008;90(10): 1278–83.

35. Sharma S, Vassan U, Bhamra M. Metal-on-metal total hip joint replacement: a minimum follow-up of five years. Hip Int 2007;17(2):70–7.

36. Saito S, Ryu J, Ishii T, et al. Midterm results of Metasul metal-on-metal total hip arthroplasty. J Arthropl 2006;21(8):1105–10.

37. McLaughlin J, Lee K. Total hip arthroplasty with an uncemented femoral component. Excellent results at ten-year follow-up. J Bone Joint Surg Br 1997; 79(6):900–7.

38. Sinha R, Dungy B, Yeon H. Primary total hip arthroplasty with a proximally porous-coated femoral stem. J Bone Joint Surgery Am 2004;86(6):1254–61.

39. Tindall A, James K, Slack R, et al. Long-term follow-up of a hydroxyapatite ceramic-coated threaded cup: an analysis of survival and fixation at up to 15 years. J Arthrop 2007;22(8):1079–82.

40. Duffy GP, Berry DJ, Rowland C, et al. Primary uncemented total hip arthroplasty in patients <40 years old: 10- to 14-year results using first-generation proximally porous-coated implants. J Arthroplasty 2001;16(8 Suppl 1):140–4.

41. Garcia-Cimbrelo E, Cruz-Pardos A, Madero R, et al. Total Hip Arthroplasty with Use of the Cementless Zweymuller Alloclassic System: a ten to thirteen-year follow-up study. J Bone Joint Surg Am 2003; 85-A(2):296–303.

42. Mallory T, Lombardi AJ, Leith J, et al. Minimal 10-year results of a tapered cementless femoral component in total hip arthroplasty. J Arthroplasty 2001;16(8 Suppl 1):49–54.

43. Richards C, Duncan C, Bassam A, et al. Femoral revision hip arthroplasty a comparison of two stem designs. Clin Orthop Relat Res 2010;468(2): 491–6.

44. McGrath M, Marker DR, Seyler T, et al. Surface replacement is comparable to primary total hip arthroplasty. Clin Orthop Relat Res 2009;467: 94–100.

45. Ball S, Le Duff M, Amstutz H. Early results of conversion of a failed femoral component in hip resurfacing arthroplasty. J Bone Joint Surg Am 2007;89: 735–41.

46. Daniel J, Ziaee H, Kamali A, et al. Ten-year results of a double-heat-treated metal-on-metal hip resurfacing. J Bone Joint Surg Br 2010;92(1):20–7.

47. Garbuz D, Tanzer M, Greidanus N, et al. The John Charnley Award: metal-on-metal hip resurfacing versus large-diameter head metal-on-metal total hip arthroplasty: a randomized clinical trial. Clin Orthop Relat Res 2010;468(2):318–25.

48. Lavigne M, Therrien M, Nantel J, et al. The John Charnley Award: the functional outcome of hip resurfacing and large-head THA is the same: a randomized, double-blind Study. Clin Orthop Relat Res 2010;468(2):326–36.

49. Lavigne M, Masse V, Girard J, et al. Return to sport after hip resurfacing or total hip arthroplasty: a randomized study. Rev Chir Orthop Reparatrice Appar Mot 2008;94(4):361–7.

50. Pollard T, Baker R, Eastaugh-Waring S, et al. Treatment of the young active patient with osteoarthritis of the hip. A five- to seven-year comparison of hybrid total hip arthroplasty and metal-on-metal resurfacing. J Bone Joint Surg Br 2006;88(5):592–600.

51. Vendittoli P, Ganapathi M, Roy A, et al. A comparison of clinical results of hip resurfacing arthroplasty and 28 mm metal on metal total hip arthroplasty: a randomised trial with 3-6 years follow-up. Hip Int 2010; 20(1):1–13.

52. Pocock N, Eisman J, Gwinn T, et al. Muscle strength, physical fitness, and weight but not age predict femoral neck bone mass. J Bone Miner Res 1989; 4(3):441–8.

53. Amstutz H, Su E, Le Duff M, et al. Are there benefits to one- versus two-stage procedures in bilateral hip resurfacing? Clin Orthop Relat Res 2010. [Epub ahead of print].

54. Prosser G, Yates P, Wood D, et al. Outcome of primary resurfacing hip replacement: evaluation of risk factors for early revision. Acta Orthop 2010; 468(2):382–91.

55. Nunley R, Zhu J, Brooks P, et al. The learning curve for adopting hip resurfacing among hip specialists. Clin Orthop Relat Res 2010;468(2):382–91.

56. O'Neill M, Beaule P, Bin Nasser A, et al. Canadian academic experience with metal-on-metal hip resurfacing. Bull NYU Hosp Jt Dis 2009;67(2):128–31.

57. Witjes S, Smolders J, Beaulé P, et al. Learning from the learning curve in total hip resurfacing: a radiographic analysis. Arch Orthop Trauma Surg 2009; 129(10):1293–9.

58. Amstutz H. Indications for metal-on-metal hybrid hip resurfacing. In: Amstutz HC, editor. Hip resurfacing: principles, indications, technique and results. Philadelphia: Elsevier; 2008. p. 95–102.

Comparison of Functional Results of Hip Resurfacing and Total Hip Replacement: A Review of the Literature

Andrew J. Shimmin, MBBS, FAorthA, FRACS*,
Jon V. Baré, MBBS, FAorthA, FRACS

KEYWORDS

- Total hip • Replacement • Resurfacing • Arthroplasty
- Function

Total hip arthroplasty (THA) has long been considered the treatment of choice for osteoarthritis of the hip in older patients. This procedure results in consistently good outcomes in function and risk for revision in this patient demographic. However, the same procedure performed in young, active patients results in an increased rate of revision and less favorable outcome of those revision proceedures.[1–4]

Modern metal-on-metal hip resurfacing arthroplasty (HRA), despite having a higher overall rate of revision[1,5] and less evidence-based literature supporting its use in all demographics, is perceived by patients as being a safer, more effective treatment that results in a greater range of motion than THA.[6] In the literature, HRA is often described as an appropriate treatment of hip osteoarthritis in young, active patients.[7–9] In Australia, 50% of HRA is performed in patients who are less than 55 years of age.[1]

The active lifestyle of younger patients places additional stresses on hip prostheses for a prolonged period of time that are not encountered in older patients. Furthermore, young active patients are less tolerant of compromised function and, therefore, selection of an appropriate prosthesis that provides good functionality and durability is critical in these patients.[2] Data that compare the functional results of HRA and THA across different patient demographics and activity levels give surgeons the ability to make adequately informed, patient-based decisions regarding prosthesis selection.

We have examined the literature to prepare a review of published studies that compare the functional results of THA and HRA. Specific outcomes such as range of motion, activity level, groin pain, patient satisfaction, and restoration of normal hip anatomy and gait are addressed separately.

METHODS

The authors systematically reviewed the literature on hip resurfacing outcomes using the PubMed bibliographic database. An initial search was performed to identify all articles that might be relevant to the review by collecting all entries with the keywords "hip resurfacing," "resurfacing

The authors have nothing to disclose.
Melbourne Orthopaedic Group, 33 The Avenue, Windsor, Victoria 3181, Australia
* Corresponding author.
E-mail address: ashimmin@optusnet.com.au

Orthop Clin N Am 42 (2011) 143–151
doi:10.1016/j.ocl.2010.12.007

arthroplasty," "hip resurfacing versus total hip" and "functional outcome hip resurfacing." The initial keyword search yielded 713 articles. The abstracts of these articles were searched to determine whether they were suitable for inclusion in this review. In examining the references generated by this process, articles were selected that discussed the functional outcome of HRA compared with the functional outcome of conventional total hip replacement, with preference given to studies in which patients were matched for age, gender, and preoperative function. Of the 713 articles found using the keyword search, 46 articles were selected for further evaluation. No preference was given to articles in which a specific femoral head size was used for either HRA or conventional THA. Review articles and the bibliographies of each reference were also searched to find additional articles that appeared relevant.

RESULTS
Range of Motion

Range of motion (ROM) is particularly important for younger patients who wish to return to a highly active lifestyle following joint replacement. Limited ROM may be a consequence of impingement, which may cause subluxation and hence high levels of wear and early failure.[10]

In vitro studies including both cadaver and computer simulation studies consistently show that HRA results in reduced ROM when compared with conventional THA. Bengs and colleagues[11] evaluated 3 contemporary hip resurfacing systems and compared 20 different movements (10 with zero femoral anteversion, and 10 with 20 degrees femoral anteversion) with those of 5 conventional hip replacement systems. Overall, the hip resurfacing systems resulted in less ROM than the conventional THA systems, with the conventional THA having significantly more ROM in 12 of the 20 movements tested. The summed mean arcs of motion in the sagittal, coronal, and axial planes for the HRA group were 135, 78, and 115 degrees, compared with 174, 87, and 150 degrees for the zero anteversion group, and 158, 90, and 147 degrees for the groups with 20 degrees of anteversion. These findings are consistent with those of Kluess and colleagues,[10] who showed that ROM for 8 designs of hip resurfacing prosthesis tested in 3 different leg positions were on average 31 to 48 degrees less than for conventional hip replacements using a 32-mm head diameter. In both studies, neck-on-cup impingement was the cause of the observed reduction in ROM. Incavo and colleagues[12] attempted to eliminate all patient-related variables by using a combination of cadaver/computer simulation. The investigators found that, with controlled patient variables, THA was able to restore normal ROM more effectively than HRA. Surface replacement showed minor deficits in extension and significant reductions in flexion and internal rotation at 90° compared with the natural hip. The investigators concluded that decreased ROM for the HRA group was attributed to a smaller head-neck ratio or head-neck offset at points of impingement.

The translation of the results from these in vitro studies to the clinical situation is limited because they do not accurately mimic the complex nature of the in vivo implanted hip. Differences may be expected because of variation in hip anatomy and musculotendinous attachments, as well as subtle differences in surgical approach. Furthermore, fear of instability for hips treated with THA and the benefits of complete capsular release in HRA that overcomes preoperative soft tissue contracture may also cause discrepancies between the results of in vitro and in vivo studies.

Clinical studies report that the ROM for THA and HRA is similar or even better for HRA (**Table 1**). Vail and colleagues,[13] in a study of 52 patients (57 hips) with resurfacing and 84 patients (93 hips) with cementless THAs, found that, after controlling for age, gender, and preoperative differences, the resurfacing group had significantly higher ROM scores than did the cementless THA group after a mean follow-up of 3 years. However, Lavigne and colleagues,[14] in a single-blind randomized study using digital photography of hip motion, failed to find a difference between patients assigned to the HRA group and the THA group at 1-year follow-up. In this study, patient demographics and preoperative ROM were similar. Le Duff and colleagues[15] also found no difference in ROM between patients treated bilaterally, with an HRA on one side and a conventional THA in the contralateral limb to control patient variability. The investigators reported that the ROM for both implant types was consistent with the ROM seen in normal, undiseased hips. It is possible that, although THA can result in significantly greater ROM in the laboratory setting, this increased ROM is unable to be achieved in patients with normal to average flexibility, thereby resulting in a similar clinical ROM for THA and HRA.

In summary, although the geometry of hip resurfacing components may limit their ROM in the laboratory setting, clinically patients may expect to achieve equivalent, if not better, ROM following HRA. If patients do experience a decreased ROM as a consequence of impingement, then subluxation and edge loading may occur, which can lead to a higher wear rate and early failure.

Table 1
Ranges of motion reported in the literature for patients treated with HRA and conventional THA

Study	No. of Patients	Mean Follow-up (mo)	Type of Evaluation	HRA	THA	P Value
Lavigne et al,[37] 2010	24 HRA 24 THA	12	Total arc of motion	204.2	196.5	>.05
			Arc of rotation	47.7	44.3	
			Flexion-extension arc	118.1	120.1	
			Abduction/adduction arc	43.1	42.9	
Le Duff et al,[15] 2009	35 HRA 35 THA	88	Abduction/ adduction Angle	71 (45–85)	70 (50–95)	.6477
			Flexion arc	121 (80–140)	119 (70–140)	.4322
			Rotation arc	75 (30–115)	72 (30–110)	.5420
Vail et al,[13] 2006	52 HRA 84 THA	24	ROM score	5.0	4.8	<.001

Activity Level

Many young patients, once relieved of their arthritic pain, may return to a physically active lifestyle after hip arthroplasty.

Most clinical studies report that patients return to high levels of activity after surgery. Six out of 7 studies that compare postoperative activity levels between HRA and THA report that patients have significantly increased activity levels when treated with HRA compared with THA.[13,16–21] A summary of postoperative activity scores is presented in **Table 2**. Vail and colleagues[13] found significantly higher postoperative UCLA activity scores for patients in the HRA group[14] compared with the THA group.[13] Although the outcomes were controlled for age, gender, and preoperative clinical scores, there was variation in the demographic profile and preoperative hip score. Mont and colleagues,[17] in a comparison of 54 consecutive HRAs and 54 consecutive THAs, found significantly higher postoperative activity levels in the HRA group (see **Table 2**). In the study by Mont and colleagues, the patients were matched according to demographics and preoperative Harris hip score; however, patients were not matched according to preoperative activity level. It was subsequently found that, before surgery, patients treated with HRA had a significantly higher weighted activity score, which, given that preoperative activity level has a positive influence on functional outcome, makes interpretation of these findings challenging. Pollard and colleagues,[19] in a study comparing the outcome of hip resurfacing with THA in patients that were matched for age, gender, body mass index (BMI, calculated as weight in kilograms divided by the square of height in meters), and preoperative activity score, found higher University of California, Los Angeles (UCLA) activity scores in the resurfaced patients (see **Table 2**). Significantly more patients treated with HRA ran, participated in sport, or performed heavy manual labor than those treated with THA, a finding that is also reported by Vendittoli and colleagues[20] and Pattyn and De Smet.[18] These findings are further supported by Zywiel and colleagues,[21] who evaluated patients that were matched in age, gender, BMI, and preoperative activity level. Pre- and postoperative activity levels were measured using a weighted activity questionnaire. At follow-up, the resurfacing patients had a significantly higher mean weighted activity score than those treated with THA (10.0 points, range 1.0–27.5 points, compared with 5.3 points, range 0–12.0 points).

In the studies described here, the postoperative clinical scores such as Harris hip score, satisfaction score and pain score were similar between patients treated with HRA and those treated with THA, despite significant differences in postoperative activity level. This finding highlights the lack of sensitivity of common scoring systems caused by a ceiling effect that makes it difficult to distinguish between patients at the upper end of the scoring scale.[22] Furthermore, it highlights the value of weighted activity scores in evaluating postoperative functional outcome, a sentiment that is shared by Zywiel and colleagues.[21]

Groin Pain

A critical aspect in achieving a good functional outcome is the correct positioning of both the femoral and acetabular components, which is more challenging in HRA. More specifically, the difficulties encountered during implantation of the acetabular component can result in prominence of the acetabular component anteriorly, which

Table 2
Functional outcome scores reported in the literature for patients treated with HRA and conventional THA

Study	No. of Patients	Mean Follow-up (mo)	WOMAC		OHS		HHS		UCLA/Activity Score	
			Preop	Postop	Preop	Postop	Preop	Postop	Preop	Postop
Mont et al,[17] 2009	54 HRA	39 (24–60)	—	—	—	—	52 (33–71)	90 (50–100)	3 (0–15)[a]	11.5 (0–32)[a]
	54 THA	39 (24–56)					50 (32–73)	91 (62–100)	2 (0–6)[a]	7 (0–21)[a]
Killampalli et al,[16] 2009	58 HRA	5 y (4–7)	—	—	44.4 (31–57)	16.6 (12–31)	—	—	4.2 (1–8)	6.7 (3–10)
	58 THA				46.1 (16–60)	18.8 (12–45)			3.4 (1–7)	5.8 (3–10)
Hall et al,[27] 2009	33 HRA	6	—	—	38.1 (36.0–40.2)	18.6 (16.3–20.8)	—	—	—	—
	99 THA				41.7 (40.1–43.4)	21.5 (19.2–23.1)				
Vendittoli et al,[20] 2010	109 HRA	2 y	52.7 ± 15.4	5.7 ± 8.6	—	—	—	—	—	7.5 ± 1.8
	100 THA		54.4 ± 18.3	9.0 ± 11.9						7.1 ± 1.6
Sandiford et al,[39] 2010	141 HRA	19.2	45.9	6.1 (0–56)	37 (13–57)	15 (12–35)	54.1 (7–97)	96.8 (59–100)	3	9
	141 THA	13.4	50.9 (3–96)	5 (0–39)	41.1 (16–75)	14.8 (12–33)	46.4 (7–87)	95.8 (65–100)	2	9
Lavigne et al,[37] 2010	24 HRA	12	46.5 (26–79)	3.0 (0–12)	—	—	—	—	—	8.0 (5–10)
	24 THA		54.3 (30–80)	2.7 (0–16)						8.3 (6–10)
Rahman et al,[40] 2010	329 HRA	6.6 y (5–9.2)	47.9 (5–96)	6.9 (0–58)	38.3 (16–60)	15.9 (12–46)	51.3 (7–91)	94.3 (24–100)	4.7 (1–9)	7.5 (3–10)
Pollard et al,[19] 2006	54 HRA	61 (52–71)	—	—	—	15.9 (12–42)	—	—	9 (6–10)	8.4 (4–10)
	54 THA	80 (42–120)				18.5 (12–41)			8.9 (6–10)	6.8 (3–10)
Fowble et al,[41] 2009	50 HRA	38 (24–50)	—	—	—	—	46 (25–59)	97 (81–100)	4.2 (2–7)	8.2 (4–10)
	44 THA	30 (24–48)					52 (30–73)	96 (66–100)	3.6 (2–7)	5.9 (3–10)
Zywiel et al,[21] 2009	33 HRA	42 (25–68)	—	—	—	—	52 (28–71)	91 (32–100)	2.1 (0–6)[a]	10 (1–27.5)[a]
	33 THA	45 (24–67)					49 (20–69)	90 (50–100)	2.3 (0–6)[a]	5.3 (0–12)[a]

Abbreviations: HHS, Harris hip score; OHS, Oxford hip score; Postop, after surgery; Preop, before surgery; UCLA, University of California, Los Angeles; WOMAC, Western Ontario and McMaster Universities Osteoarthritis Index.

[a] Adapted scoring system previously used for total knee arthroplasty.[17]

Data from Mont MA, Marker DR, Smith JM, et al. Resurfacing is comparable to total hip arthroplasty at short-term follow-up. Clin Orthop Relat Res 2009;467:66.

has been associated with groin pain caused by irritation of the Iliopsoas tendon. In addition, failure to recognize and treat underlying femoroacetabular impingement lesions can result in ongoing impingement of the femoral neck in flexion.[23,24]

There are currently few studies that compare the incidence of groin pain between HRA and THA. Bin Nasser and colleagues[25] evaluated the incidence of groin pain after metal-on-metal hip resurfacing for 116 patients with a mean follow-up of 26 months. Twenty-one patients (18%) reported persistent groin pain, with a mean pain score of 5.19 out of 10. Deep anterior groin pain that was aggravated by activity was reported in all of these patients. In patients reporting groin pain, 52% required analgesics and 57% reported that the pain limited their activities. Although patients reporting groin pain improved after surgery, their improvement was less than in those without groin pain.

A similar incidence of groin pain was reported recently by Bartelt and colleagues[26] following a retrospective review of 282 hips treated with either HRA or THA at a mean follow-up of 14 months. Those treated with a conventional metal-on-polyethylene THA bearing reported a 7% incidence of groin pain compared with 18% if treated by metal-on-metal HRA. Of the patients receiving a metal-on-metal THA, 15% reported groin pain. The investigators suggest that the higher incidence of groin pain in the HRA group may have been a consequence of hypersensitivity to the metal-on-metal bearings or greater impingement of the psoas tendon. In this study, younger patients more frequently reported pain; however, a gender association was not found because of the large number of male patients enrolled in this study. The investigators propose that the higher activity and expectation levels in younger patients may make them more likely to report pain after surgery.

The incidence of groin pain reported for HRA in these 2 studies is considerably higher than that reported for conventional metal-on-polyethylene THA.[24] It should be noted that in neither of these two studies was reference made to implant choice, surgical approach or implant orientation. Although these issues are important in all arthroplasty, they are particularly important in resurfacing arthroplasty.

Patient Satisfaction, Quality of Life, and Postoperative Pain

There are several validated scoring systems such as Harris hip score, Oxford hip score, Western Ontario and McMaster Universities Osteoarthritis Index (WOMAC) and UCLA activity scores that are used to evaluate the functional outcome of HRA and THA. Although these scoring systems provide useful information regarding many aspects of functional outcome, they are limited in their ability to measure satisfaction from the perspective of the patient.

Several studies report survey-based measures of patient satisfaction, and, although differences in the methods of measuring satisfaction vary between studies, the data provide us with some insight into the patient-perceived outcome of hip replacement. In general, studies report high patient satisfaction levels for both HRA and THA. Even studies in which no difference in satisfaction was observed between patients treated with THA and HRA, overall satisfaction reported was high for both treatments.[13,17,21]

Hall and colleagues[27] measured patient satisfaction in a case-matched control study and found that patients treated with HRA were more likely to report excellent or very good pain relief at 6 months, and also reported better heavy lifting ability at 6 months. Overall, both HRA and THA resulted in similar, very high patient satisfaction. This study also found that good preoperative function had a positive effect on postoperative satisfaction. Using an 11-point Likert scale, Mont and colleagues[17] also observed that postoperative pain was similar following HRA and THA, with both procedures resulting in low pain scores of 1.4 and 1.6 for HRA and THA respectively.

Vendittoli and colleagues[28] also found high satisfaction rates for both HRA and THA, with 99% of patients in both the HRA and THA groups reporting that they were satisfied or very satisfied with their procedure. Pain scores measured in this study were also similar between the 2 treatment groups. The only difference found was that a higher percentage of HRA patients experienced pain on rising from a chair (21% compared with 8% for THAs) at the earliest time point of 6 months. In a comparison of the return to function following HRA and THA, Stulberg and colleagues[29] also found a trend for resurfacing patients to have increased pain during the early postoperative period (6 weeks). However, by 24 months there was no difference in pain level between patients having undergone HRA or THA.

Quality of life scores measured by Pollard and colleagues[19] were better for patients treated with HRA. Mean EuroQol 5 part questionaire (EQ-5D) scores were 0.78 and 0.9 for THA and HRA respectively. Similarly, mean EuroQol visual analogue scale (EQ-VAS) scores were 69.3 and 82.3 for THA and HRA respectively. However, there was no preoperative evaluation of hip score in this study and it is therefore possible that patients in the HRA group had better preoperative hip function, which, as was found in the study by Hall and colleagues,[27] is a positive contributor to postoperative outcome. In contrast, a recent study by Garbuz and colleagues[30] found no difference in quality of life as measured by Short form health survey-12 questions (SF-12), WOMAC, and Quality of Life Outcome Index 5 Questions (PAT 5-D) scores, nor did they find any difference in UCLA activity score. However, this study compared HRA with a large-head metal-on-metal THA.

In summary, studies report high patient satisfaction for both THA and HRA. This satisfaction is most likely the result of high postoperative activity level and good pain relief. However, additional factors, such as patient perception and expectation, are also likely to contribute to the observed satisfaction scores.

Functional Scores

A summary of the functional scores from 9 recent studies that report the outcome of HRA compared with THA is provided in **Table 2**. The functional scores most frequently reported include Oxford hip score, Harris hip score, SF-12 scores, WOMAC, and UCLA activity scores. The functional scores reported are consistent between these studies. In 8 of the 9 studies, the HRA group had better preoperative function than the THA. All of the 9 studies reported an improvement in functional score after surgery for both HRA and THA; however, functional scores were consistently similar between the 2 procedures. Factors that are likely to influence functional outcome include gender, age, and preoperative function.

Restoration of Normal Hip Anatomy and Gait

It is important to restore normal hip biomechanics during the hip arthroplasty procedure to maximize ROM and to avoid leg length and gait abnormalities, dislocation, and increased wear, all of which can contribute to implant failure and ultimately patient dissatisfaction.

There are a small number of studies that have directly compared the outcome of THA and HRA in terms of restoration of normal hip anatomy and limb length. The data from these studies are contradictory, which, given their small number, makes it difficult to draw firm conclusions regarding their outcomes.

Three studies present similar results. Girard and colleagues,[31] in a radiographic analysis of 49 hip resurfacings and 55 THAs, found that femoral offset and limb length were increased when compared with the contralateral limb following THA. In contrast, femoral offset and limb length

were reduced following HRA. Limb length inequality was restored in 86% of resurfacings compared with only 60% of THA. The investigators concluded that biomechanical reconstruction of the femur is more reproducible with HRA. Ahmad and colleagues[32] presented similar findings in a comparison of femoral offset and limb length between 28 THAs and 28 HRAs. THA resulted in increased femoral offset, whereas HRA resulted in reduced change in limb length. Also presenting similar findings, Robb and colleagues[33] concluded that, although there was no difference in restoration of leg lengths, HRA more accurately restores femoral and total offset than cemented THA. In contrast, Loughead and colleagues[34] found a greater increase in femoral length following HRA combined with a greater reduction in femoral offset, and concluded that HRA does not restore limb length or offset more accurately than THA.

Gait analysis has been used in an attempt to differentiate any functional differences between HRA and THA. Some gait analysis studies provide evidence to suggest that HRA results in equivalent or better walking speed, abductor moment, and extensor moment than THA.

Mont and colleagues[35] compared walking speed, abductor, and extensor moments between 15 patients treated with THA, 15 patients treated with HRA, and 10 patients with untreated osteoarthritis of the hip after a mean follow-up of 13 months, and found that patients treated with HRA were able to walk significantly faster than patients treated with THA and had gait parameters that were closer to normal. Shrader and colleagues[36] reported similar findings in a pilot study evaluating walking speed and stair negotiation in 7 patients treated with THA, 7 treated with HRA and 7 normal controls. Patients treated with HRA had more normal patterns of movement with greater improvement in hip abduction and extension moments than patients treated with THA. Stair negotiation was also improved in the HRA group. Lavigne and colleagues[37] reported equivalent gait speed at both normal walking speed and fast walking speed for 48 patients treated with THA and 48 patients treated with HRA when evaluated at a mean of 14 months. Evaluation of postural balance was also similar between the groups. Patients in both treatment groups reached most control group values by 3 months after surgery. Similar findings were presented by Shimmin and colleagues[38] in a comparison of patients with a postoperative Harris hip score of 100 treated with THA and HRA using the normal contralateral hip as a control. Gait at a fast walking or jogging pace, as well as abductor strength and stair climbing speed, was similar between the groups.

In summary, further studies that evaluate restoration of hip and limb anatomy and their effect on gait are necessary to be able to draw accurate conclusions on the benefits of HRA compared with THA in young, active patients. However, the limited data currently available suggest that the closer approximation of the proximal femoral anatomy combined with the conservation of proximal femoral bone stock achieved with HRA may result in a more normal gait in these patients.

SUMMARY

Hip resurfacing offers bone preservation and potential simplification of revision in young patients who are likely to outlive any contemporary implant. The findings of the studies presented in this review of the literature suggest that HRA provides equivalent, if not better, functional outcomes in well-selected patients.

There are numerous factors that affect functional outcome in patients following hip arthroplasty of any type. These factors include patient expectation, preoperative function, and general health, age, gender, and compliance with postoperative rehabilitation programs. Patients who are treated with HRA are often younger men, with better preoperative function than patients treated with THA. In addition, patients have improved expectations regarding the outcomes of HRA. Given that these factors have a positive influence on postoperative outcome, it is important for studies to match patients for age, gender, and preoperative function.

In comparison with literature describing the outcome of conventional THA alone, studies that evaluate the outcome of HRA often have a short to medium duration. Longer-term studies are necessary to determine whether the potential functional benefits of HRA in younger, active patients persist for the lifetime of the prosthesis. This consideration is of particular importance given that many patients who have had hip resurfacing are likely to outlive the prosthesis.

The increased incidence of groin pain reported in HRA highlights the importance of accurate positioning and addressing the underlying impingement disorder, which is especially important in the HRA demographic, where impingement is frequently seen as the reason for the natural joint to degenerate.

This analysis has highlighted the limited value of conventional functional scoring systems for differentiating between the functional outcomes of 2 similarly effective procedures. The development of modified scoring systems with greater sensitivity is essential to detect variation in function between procedures.

In conclusion, patients who are well selected in terms of age, gender, and proximal femoral bone stock can expect a functional outcome following HRA that is equivalent to, if not better than, THA in the short to medium term.

ACKNOWLEDGMENTS

The authors wish to thank Alexandra Pearce for assistance with the preparation of the manuscript.

REFERENCES

1. Australian Orthopaedic Association Joint Replacement Register. In annual report, 2009.
2. Eskelinen A, Remes V, Helenius I, et al. Total hip arthroplasty for primary osteoarthrosis in younger patients in the Finnish arthroplasty register. 4,661 primary replacements followed for 0–22 years. Acta Orthop 2005;76:28–41.
3. Furnes O, Lie SA, Espehaug B, et al. Hip disease and the prognosis of total hip replacements. A review of 53,698 primary total hip replacements reported to the Norwegian Arthroplasty Register 1987–99. J Bone Joint Surg Br 2001;83:579–86.
4. Malchau H, Herberts P, Ahnfelt L. Prognosis of total hip replacement in Sweden. Follow-up of 92,675 operations performed 1978–1990. Acta Orthop Scand 1993;64:497–506.
5. Corten K, MacDonald SJ. Hip resurfacing data from national joint registries: what do they tell us? What do they not tell us? Clin Orthop Relat Res 2010; 468:351–7.
6. Murphy TP, Trousdale RT, Pagnano MW, et al. Patients' perceptions of hip resurfacing arthroplasty. Orthopedics 2009;32:730.
7. Bozic KJ, Pui CM, Ludeman MJ, et al. Do the potential benefits of metal-on-metal hip resurfacing justify the increased cost and risk of complications? Clin Orthop Relat Res 2010;468:2301–12.
8. Marker DR, Strimbu K, McGrath MS, et al. Resurfacing versus conventional total hip arthroplasty-review of comparative clinical and basic science studies. Bull NYU Hosp Jt Dis 2009;67:120–7.
9. Quesada MJ, Marker DR, Mont MA. Metal-on-metal hip resurfacing: advantages and disadvantages. J Arthroplasty 2008;23:69–73.
10. Kluess D, Zietz C, Lindner T, et al. Limited range of motion of hip resurfacing arthroplasty due to unfavorable ratio of prosthetic head size and femoral neck diameter. Acta Orthop 2008;79:748–54.

11. Bengs BC, Sangiorgio SN, Ebramzadeh E. Less range of motion with resurfacing arthroplasty than with total hip arthroplasty: in vitro examination of 8 designs. Acta Orthop 2008;79:755–62.

12. Incavo SJ, Thompson MT, Gold JE, et al. Which procedure better restores intact hip range of motion: total hip arthroplasty or resurfacing? A combined cadaveric and computer simulation study. J Arthroplasty 2010. [Epub ahead of print].

13. Vail TP, Mina CA, Yergler JD, et al. Metal-on-metal hip resurfacing compares favorably with THA at 2 years followup. Clin Orthop Relat Res 2006;453: 123–31.

14. Lavigne M, Mottard S, Girard J, et al. Range of motion after hip resurfacing and THA: a single-blind randomized clinical study. Proceedings of the 75th Annual American Academy of Orthopaedic Surgeons Meeting. San Francisco, March 5–9, 2008. p. 384.

15. Le Duff MJ, Wisk LE, Amstutz HC. Range of motion after stemmed total hip arthroplasty and hip resurfacing-a clinical study. Bull NYU Hosp Jt Dis 2009; 67:177–81.

16. Killampalli VV, Kundra RK, Chaudhry F, et al. Resurfacing and uncemented arthroplasty for young hip arthritis: functional outcomes at 5 years. Hip Int 2009;19:234–8.

17. Mont MA, Marker DR, Smith JM, et al. Resurfacing is comparable to total hip arthroplasty at short-term follow-up. Clin Orthop Relat Res 2009;467:66–71.

18. Pattyn C, De Smet KA. Primary ceramic-on-ceramic total hip replacement versus metal-on-metal hip resurfacing in young active patients. Orthopedics 2008;31:1078.

19. Pollard TC, Baker RP, Eastaugh-Waring SJ, et al. Treatment of the young active patient with osteoarthritis of the hip. A five- to seven-year comparison of hybrid total hip arthroplasty and metal-on-metal resurfacing. J Bone Joint Surg Br 2006;88:592–600.

20. Vendittoli PA, Lavigne M, Roy AG, et al. A prospective randomized clinical trial comparing metal-on-metal total hip arthroplasty and metal-on-metal total hip resurfacing in patients less than 65 years old. Hip Int 2006;16(Suppl 4):73–81.

21. Zywiel MG, Marker DR, McGrath MS, et al. Resurfacing matched to standard total hip arthroplasty by preoperative activity levels - a comparison of postoperative outcomes. Bull NYU Hosp Jt Dis 2009;67:116–9.

22. Wamper KE, Sierevelt IN, Poolman RW, et al. The Harris hip score: do ceiling effects limit its usefulness in orthopedics? Acta Orthop 2010; 81:703–7.

23. Dora C, Houweling M, Koch P, et al. Iliopsoas impingement after total hip replacement: the results of non-operative management, tenotomy or acetabular revision. J Bone Joint Surg Br 2007;89:1031–5.

24. O'Sullivan M, Tai CC, Richards S, et al. Iliopsoas tendonitis a complication after total hip arthroplasty. J Arthroplasty 2007;22:166–70.

25. Bin Nasser A, Beaule PE, O'Neill M, et al. Incidence of groin pain after metal-on-metal hip resurfacing. Clin Orthop Relat Res 2010;468:392–9.

26. Bartelt RB, Yuan BJ, Trousdale RT, et al. The prevalence of groin pain after metal-on-metal total hip arthroplasty and total hip resurfacing. Clin Orthop Relat Res 2010;468:2346–56.

27. Hall DP, Srikantharajah D, Anakwe RE, et al. Patient-reported outcome following metal-on-metal resurfacing of the hip and total hip replacement. Hip Int 2009;19:245–50.

28. Venditoli PA, Ganapathi M, Roy AG, et al. A comparison of clinical results of hip resurfacing arthroplasty and 28 mm metal on metal total hip arthroplasty: a randomised trial with 3–6 years follow-up. Hip Int 2010;20:1–3.

29. Stulberg BN, Fitts SM, Bowen AR, et al. Early return to function after hip resurfacing: is it better than contemporary total hip arthroplasty? J Arthroplasty 2010;25:748–53.

30. Garbuz DS, Tanzer M, Greidanus NV, et al. The John Charnley Award: metal-on-metal hip resurfacing versus large-diameter head metal-on-metal total hip arthroplasty: a randomized clinical trial. Clin Orthop Relat Res 2010;468:318–25.

31. Girard J, Lavigne M, Venditoli PA, et al. Biomechanical reconstruction of the hip: a randomised study comparing total hip resurfacing and total hip arthroplasty. J Bone Joint Surg Br 2006;88:721–6.

32. Ahmad R, Gillespie G, Annamalai S, et al. Leg length and offset following hip resurfacing and hip replacement. Hip Int 2009;19:136–40.

33. Robb C, Harris R, O'Dwyer K, et al. Radiographic assessment of biomechanical parameters following hip resurfacing and cemented total hip arthroplasty. Hip Int 2009;19:251–6.

34. Loughead JM, Chesney D, Holland JP, et al. Comparison of offset in Birmingham hip resurfacing and hybrid total hip arthroplasty. J Bone Joint Surg Br 2005;87:163–6.

35. Mont MA, Seyler TM, Ragland PS, et al. Gait analysis of patients with resurfacing hip arthroplasty compared with hip osteoarthritis and standard total hip arthroplasty. J Arthroplasty 2007;22: 100–8.

36. Shrader MW, Bhowmik-Stoker M, Jacofsky MC, et al. Gait and stair function in total and resurfacing hip arthroplasty: a pilot study. Clin Orthop Relat Res 2009;467:1476–84.

37. Lavigne M, Therrien M, Nantel J, et al. The John Charnley Award: the functional outcome of hip resurfacing and large-head THA is the same: a randomized,

double-blind study. Clin Orthop Relat Res 2010;468: 326–36.

38. Shimmin A, Bennell K, Wrigley T, et al. Gait analysis comparison of the functional outcome of hip resurfacing and total hip replacement. Proceedings of the 75th Annual American Academy of Orthopaedic Surgeons Meeting. San Francisco, March 5–9, 2008. p. 382.

39. Sandiford NA, Muirhead-Allwood SK, Skinner JA, et al. Metal on metal hip resurfacing versus uncemented custom total hip replacement–early results. J Orthop Surg Res 2010;5:8.

40. Rahman L, Muirhead-Allwood SK, Alkinj M. What is the midterm survivorship and function after hip resurfacing? Clin Orthop Relat Res 2010;468: 3221–7.

41. Fowble VA, dela Rosa MA, Schmalzried TP. A comparison of total hip resurfacing and total hip arthroplasty - patients and outcomes. Bull NYU Hosp Jt Dis 2009;67:108–12.

Survivorship of Conserve® Plus Monoblock Metal-on-Metal Hip Resurfacing Sockets: Radiographic Midterm Results of 580 Patients

J.B. Hulst, MD[a], S.T. Ball, MD[a], G. Wu, MD[a],
Michel J. Le Duff, MA[b], R.P. Woon, MPH[b],
Harlan C. Amstutz, MD[b],*

KEYWORDS

- Conserve® Plus monoblock • Metal-on-metal
- Hip resurfacing • Arthroplasty

Reports of the durability of certain first-generation metal-on-metal total hip arthroplasty implants led to a renewed interest in this bearing couple in the 1980s.[1,2] Low wear rates associated with metal-bearing surfaces and the material's ability to withstand stresses have enabled larger head sizes required for resurfacing arthroplasty of the hip.[3] Large-diameter femoral heads continue to be attractive for total hip arthroplasty because they provide increased stability and decreased dislocation rates.[4,5] Previously, large diameter heads in metal-on-polyethylene articulations were impractical, given the unacceptable high amount of volumetric wear.[3] Over the past decade, many hip surgeons have become interested in metal-on-metal resurfacing arthroplasty for end-stage arthrosis in young active patients.

Resurfacing systems typically use press-fit, monoblock, cobalt chrome alloy acetabular sockets. These sockets differ from the modular titanium shells, which are typically used in conventional total hip replacement. Monoblock cobalt chrome cups are stiffer than their titanium counterparts and they do not allow for initial screw fixation and thus are entirely dependent on stability from a sound press-fit at initial implantation.[6,7] Furthermore, concerns have arisen because of heightened awareness of the potential for adverse local soft tissue reaction (ALTR) to metal-on-metal bearings, particularly with certain designs.[8–11]

Outcomes data on the longevity of these sockets are needed. The purpose of this study was to define the midterm survivorship and radiographic results of a cobalt chrome alloy monoblock acetabular component in patients who undergo hip resurfacing.

MATERIALS AND METHODS

A retrospective review was performed, which included the first 643 hips in 580 consecutive patients who were treated with hip resurfacing arthroplasty using the Conserve® Plus prosthesis (Wright Medical Technology, Arlington, TN, USA)

[a] Department of Orthopaedic Surgery, University of California at San Diego, Business Office 350 Dickinson Street, Suite 121, MC 8894, San Diego, CA 92103-8894, USA
[b] Joint Replacement Institute at St Vincent Medical Center, The South Mark Taper Building, 2200 West Third Street, Suite 400, Los Angeles, CA 90057, USA
* Corresponding author.
E-mail address: harlanamstutz@dochs.org

Orthop Clin N Am 42 (2011) 153–159
doi:10.1016/j.ocl.2011.01.004

between November 1996 and October 2003. The surgical technique used for implantation of the prostheses has been previously described[12] All hips were implanted with the original acetabular component, which has a constant thickness of 5 mm. The Conserve® Plus acetabular shell is made of cobalt, chromium, and molybdenum, with a porous coating of sintered beads 75 to 150 μm thick for cementless fixation (**Fig. 1**). The mean age of the patients at the time of surgery was 48.9 years (range, 14–78 years) and 75% were men. Their mean weight at the time of surgery was 83.5 kg (range, 42–164 kg) and body mass index (BMI, calculated as the weight in kilograms divided by height in meters squared) 27 (range 17–46). The causes were distributed as follows: osteoarthritis 66%, developmental dysplasia of the hip 10%, osteonecrosis 8%, trauma 8%, inflammatory diseases 3%, developmental or metabolic diseases 4%, other 1%. The patients were followed up for 4 months after surgery and then yearly. Whenever the patient could not come to the center for follow-up visits, radiographs performed in another institution were requested and a phone follow-up consultation scheduled. The senior author (H.C.A) also performed outside clinics in 20 different locations throughout the United States to reach those living outside Southern California. The radiographic review was performed by 2 experimenters (J.B.H and S.T.B) blinded to the clinical results of the patients. All immediate postoperative radiographs were analyzed for acetabular component position, including abduction angle, anteversion, presence of gaps between the acetabular cup and the reamed bone, and percent bone coverage in the frontal plane. Abduction and anteversion of the cup were measured using Ein-Bild-Röentgen-Analysis cup software, version 2003[13] and the contact patch to rim (CPR) distance[14] computed from these data. From the last follow-up films and with comparison to the immediate postoperative films, the presence and size of radiolucencies in the DeLee-Charnley[15] zones were recorded. Evidence of cup migration, pelvic osteolysis, and stress remodeling of the periacetabular bone of the pelvis were also noted. Heterotopic ossification was recorded using the grading system of Brooker and colleagues.[16] Kaplan-Meier[17] survival estimates were calculated using 2 different end points:

1. Revision for aseptic loss of acetabular component fixation.
2. Radiographic loss of acetabular fixation defined by a complete radiolucency covering all 3 De Lee-Charnley zones.

Radiolucency was used for further analysis, and Cox proportional hazard ratios were computed to identify possible risk factors specific to the durability of the acetabular component.

RESULTS

The average duration of the follow-up period was 10.4 years (range 7.1–14.0 years), and the mean radiographic follow of the series was 6.8 years (range 0.1–13.4 years). From this cohort, 482 hips had a radiographic follow-up collected during the fifth year after surgery or beyond. In this series, 45 hips underwent revision surgery at a mean time to revision of 61.6 months (range 1–139 months). However, the reason for revision was a loss of acetabular component fixation in only 5 hips revised at a mean of 75.2 months (range 2–120 months): At 5, 8, 9 and 10 years, 4 acetabular components loosened, and 1 component protruded through the medial acetabular wall 4 days after surgery.[18] Of these hips, 3 were revised to a conventional THR, whereas 2 were maintained as hip resurfacings by insertion of a new cup of greater outside diameter (**Fig. 2**).

The Kaplan-Meier survival estimate of the acetabular component was 99.6% at 5 years (95% confidence interval, 98.6%–99.9%) and 98.3% at 10 years (95% confidence interval, 95.5%–99.4%) when revision for loss of acetabular fixation was used as end point. In addition, 5 hips showed complete radiolucencies covering

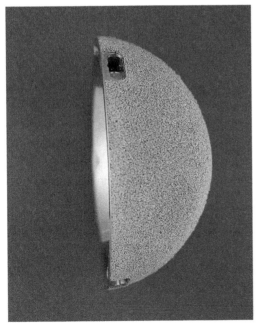

Fig. 1. Conserve® Plus original acetabular component.

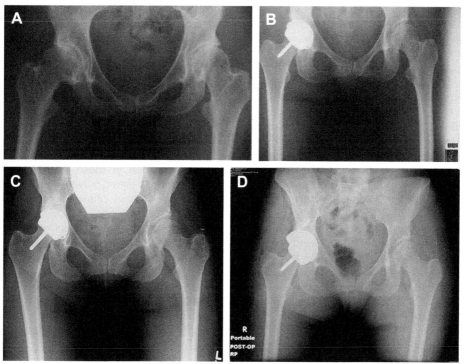

Fig. 2. (*A*) Anteroposterior preoperative radiograph of a 42-year-old woman with osteoarthritis of the right hip secondary to congenital hip dysplasia. At the time of surgery, the acetabulum was severely dysplastic, and there was erosion with cyst formation anteriorly. (*B*) On postoperative day 3, an anteroposterior radiograph shows good fixation of the metal-on-metal surface replacement (outer diameter [OD] 52–42 mm inner diameter [ID]). (*C*) Anteroposterior radiograph at 100.2 months after operation, suggesting excellent fixation. There is a dense sclerotic reaction in the acetabulum superior region to the component, which progressed over a 6-year period. (*D*) Immediate anteroposterior radiograph after revision surgery. The original femoral component remained, and the acetabular cup was revised to a Conserve® Total Superfix cup (OD 56–42 mm ID) with 2 superior fixation screws. The leg lengths are approximately equal. The patient is doing well 2 years after revision.

the 3 De Lee-Charnley zones around the cup at a mean follow-up time of 115.9 months (range, 94–127 months). Using the time to radiographic failure of these hips and the hips revised for acetabular loss of fixation as end point (**Fig. 3**), the Kaplan-Meier survival estimate of the acetabular component was 99.6% at 5 years (95% confidence interval, 98.6%–99.9%) and 97.6% at 10 years (95% confidence interval, 94.6%–98.9%).

The mean cup abduction angle was 43.5° (range 16°–72°). The mean anteversion angle of the cup was 17.4° (range 2°–51°). The mean CPR distance was 14.5 mm (range 1–25 mm), and in 79 hips, the CPR distance was less than 10 mm. Acetabular cup coverage was complete in 60.8% of the hips, ranging from 70% to 100%. All hips included, radiolucencies were visible in zone 1 for 19 cups (including 2 radiolucencies 2 mm thick), in zone 2 for 22 cups (including 4 radiolucencies 2 mm thick), and in zone 3 for 36 cups (including 6 radiolucencies 2 mm thick). Radiolucencies in multiple zones were seen in 15 cups (2.3%), including

9 cups (4 revised) with radiolucencies in all 3 zones (which were included in the second survivorship analysis). Small amounts of cup migration (≤2 mm) were observed in 7 cups (1.0%). Small

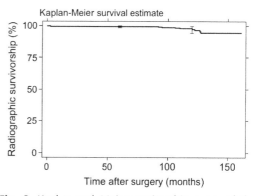

Fig. 3. Kaplan and Meier survivorship curve of the Conserve® Plus acetabular component. The time to aseptic radiographic failure was used as end point. The 95% confidence intervals are shown at 5 and 10 years.

pelvic osteolytic lesions were suspected in 15 hips (2.3%). Brooker grade III heterotopic ossification was seen in 25 hips (3.9%) and Brooker grade IV in 6 hips (0.9%).

Postoperative gaps were observed in 30 cups (4.7%) in zone 1 (4 of 2 mm or more), 118 cups (18.4%) in zone 2 (35 of ≥2 mm), and 7 cups (1.1%) in zone 3 (2 of ≥2 mm). All postoperative gaps filled in within 36 months, except in 8 hips; 4 cups settled into the original gap and appeared stable, whereas 3 showed a fibrous fixation at first follow-up. One cup was revised at 36 months for sepsis. There was no association of the presence of a gap on the postoperative radiograph and the occurrence of cup aseptic loosening.

Young age (hazard ratio 0.942, $P = .022$), low BMI (hazard ratio 0.816, $P = .027$), and low CPR distance (hazard ratio 0.848, $P = .037$) were identified as risk factors for a higher rate of cup failure to osseointegrate or subsequent loss of fixation.

DISCUSSION

This study highlights the excellent radiographic survivorship profile of the Conserve® Plus, monoblock, cobalt chrome alloy acetabular component (**Fig. 4**). Based on this series, overall acetabular component survivorship at 10-year follow-up, with the end point defined as radiographic loosening of the shell is 97.6%. This survivorship is roughly in line with survivorship reported for contemporary cementless titanium acetabular components used with stemmed total hip replacements.

Della Valle and colleagues[19] recently described the 20-year survivorship for uncemented Harris-Galante titanium shells with metal on conventional polyethylene bearing couples. When failure was defined as aseptic loosening of the acetabular component, these sockets had a 99% survivorship at 15 years and 96% at 20 years. In a similar study, Engh and colleagues[20] described the long-term results at a single institution in more than 4000 primary total hip arthroplasties using hemispheric porous coated cups. With acetabular component aseptic loosening as the end point, 15-year survivorship was reported as 94.7% for spiked cups, 98.4% for press-fit cups with screws, and 100% for press-fit cups without screws. The results of both of these studies are quite impressive given that implantation in these series predated the advent of cross-linked polyethylene.

The radiographic observations in cups that progressed to aseptic loosening were noted. Previous descriptions of radiographic osteolysis and loosening associated with titanium shells and polyethylene liners include voluminous or "ballooning" lytic defects of the ilium and ischium, which occurs and progresses late after initial ingrowth.[21] The authors' series lacked these radiographic findings. Instead, the acetabuli in the majority of the loosened cups were noted to have small lucent areas in all DeLee/Charnley zones. Increased radiographic density was sometimes noted in the adjacent acetabular bone. In 1 case, loosening was difficult to detect and was associated with minimal appreciable radiographic findings. Other imaging modalities, such as bone scan, may be indicated for diagnosis in symptomatic patients with minimal radiographic findings. There is possibility that the series may contain other loose cups yet to be identified.

The material properties of these monoblock cobalt chrome cups differ to some degree from their titanium counterparts. Cobalt chromium alloy has a higher modulus of elasticity than titanium, rendering it a stiffer material. In theory, the increased modulus mismatch between the

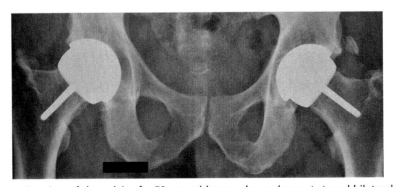

Fig. 4. Anteroposterior view of the pelvis of a 50-year-old man who underwent staged bilateral procedures for osteoarthritis of the hips. The left hip is shown 10 years after resurfacing using the 5 mm Conserve® Plus shell and the right hip 5 years after resurfacing with the subsequent 3.5 mm acetabular component. Both hips show perfect osseointegration of the cups.

monoblock cobalt chrome cup and the interfacing cortical and cancellous bone might predispose to greater amounts of micromotion and less bony ingrowth. The low rate of radiographic migration and aseptic loosening shown in the present study may indicate that this concern is unfounded. Still, it is unknown whether the failures in this series represent loosening that progresses after a period of initial ingrowth and stability (as seen with osteolysis) or failure of initial ingrowth from the outset with only fibrous fixation that eventually breaks down. The different radiographic appearance of the loose monoblock cobalt chrome cup as compared with a loose titanium shell with osteolysis may represent a different pathophysiologic process that may be a function of these different material properties and a different biologic response to the wear debris that is generated.

One of the more interesting findings in this study is the presence and fate of gaps behind the acetabular component from incomplete seating of the cup at the time of implantation. This finding is not uncommon with these monoblock shells. There are no screw holes and no dome hole. Therefore, there is no direct visual cue at the time of implantation to be absolutely certain that the cup is totally seated. Furthermore, the stiffness of the material and the excellent quality of the bone of the typical resurfacing candidate may predispose to incomplete seating during insertion. Nevertheless, in the current series, despite approximately 20% of patients being noted as having some gap, with approximately 5% of the gaps larger than 2 mm, none of these cups progressed to aseptic loosening, and almost all gaps filled in radiographically. This finding suggests that as long as a stable rim fit is obtained, the cup should remain stable and ingrown. This finding has been reported with titanium shells as well. Roth and colleagues[22] described an 18% occurrence of zone 2 gaps on immediately postoperative radiographs in anatomical medullary locking Total Hip System (Depuy orthopaedics Inc, Warsaw, IN, USA) cups placed without screw fixation, and Udomkiat and colleagues[23] reported a 34% incidence of very small gaps behind porous coated titanium cups on initial postoperative radiographs. In both of these reports, all cups with initial gaps remained stable, and there was no association with aseptic loosening similar to the findings reported in the current report.

The literature is sparse with survivorship studies of other monoblock cobalt chrome sockets. Although several studies detail the midterm outcomes for hip resurfacing arthroplasty, none specifically examine the survivorship of the acetabular implant. Survivorship analysis of the cup is important in the selection of the procedure and prosthesis and should also be considered in the event of a revision of a failed resurfacing. To maintain the conservative paradigm of resurfacing, it is intuitive to consider retaining a well-fixed and well-positioned socket and using a femoral head from the same manufacturer that matches the inner diameter of the existing shell. The favorable results and survivorship reported in the current study suggest that the acetabular component can be retained provided that it is well-positioned, well-fixed, and free of macroscopic damage. In fact, in this current series, there are 18 hips included that still have their original acetabular component after being converted to a total hip for femoral-sided failure of the resurfacing.[24] None of these shells have gone on to failure after first articulating with a resurfaced head and then articulating with a large head on a total hip stem.

The association of low CPR distance and aseptic loosening of the acetabular component suggests that the computation of this variable may have predicting value on not only the potential for increased wear of the components[14] but also the mechanical behavior of the cementless sockets and its bonding to the host acetabulum. A reduced CPR distance means that the application of the joint reaction force is directed on a more peripheral aspect of the cup, creating a potential debonding of the cup on the opposite side of the component. The gradual increase in number of radiolucencies observed from zones 1 to zone 3 further suggests this hypothesis.

Several shortcomings of this study may be considered. The authors' study is retrospective in nature, and the studied cohort did not have a control group, thereby risking the overstatement of the results. However, the main material of investigation in this study was the anteroposterior pelvis radiograph, which was collected on all cases preoperatively, immediately postoperatively, and serially until the last follow-up. In addition, the abundance of comparable data available in the literature related to conventional total hip arthroplasty provided sufficient information to assess the results of this series. Perhaps most importantly, the present study did not report specific outcome measurements such as pain or function scores. However, clinical scores do not allow to differentiate between symptoms attributable to the femoral component, the acetabular component, or systemic diseases And the scope of the authors' study was limited to the performance of the acetabular component. Also, the lack of correlation between radiographic results and clinical outcomes is unlikely to have led to an underappreciation of problems with the acetabular sockets because radiographs usually show deterioration long before the symptoms appear.

Reports of ALTRs[25] with metal bearing hip arthroplasties and resurfacings have appeared in the orthopaedic literature over the past decade.[10,11,26] The authors' study did not specifically investigate this potential mode of failure, but till now, the number of identified ALTR II (fluid or solid mass) (see the article by Amstutz and colleagues elsewhere in this issue for further exploration of this topic) in the present series is 6 (0.9%). This prevalence is very low in comparison with the rates reported in several studies[27] despite a calculated CPR distance of less than 10 mm in 79 hips (12.3%).

Overall, the results suggest that reliable and durable midterm to long-term outcomes may be expected with the use of the Conserve® Plus monoblock, metal-on-metal bearing, cobalt-chromium acetabular cup. Although some surgeons have questioned the overall safety of this articulation in young and active patients with advanced hip arthrosis, there are few satisfactory arthroplasty options, and all available resurfacing modalities use a large head metal articulation. Further long-term studies will be helpful in determining the eventual outcomes of resurfacing arthroplasty, in comparison to conventional THA with other bearing materials, and addressing concerns related to the safety of metal-on-metal articulations.

REFERENCES

1. McKellop H, Park SH, Chiesa R, et al. In vivo wear of three types of metal on metal hip prostheses during two decades of use. Clin Orthop Relat Res 1996;(Suppl 329):S128–340.
2. Schmalzried TP, Peters PC, Maurer BT, et al. Long-duration metal-on-metal total hip arthroplasties with low wear of the articulating surfaces. J Arthroplasty 1996;11(3):322–31.
3. Sieber HP, Rieker CB, Kottig P. Analysis of 118 second-generation metal-on-metal retrieved hip implants. J Bone Joint Surg Br 1999;81(1):46–50.
4. Amstutz H, Le Duff M, Beaulé P. Prevention and treatment of dislocation after total hip replacement using large diameter balls. Clin Orthop 2004; 429(12):108–16.
5. Peters C, McPherson E, Jackson J, et al. Reduction in early dislocation rate with large-diameter femoral heads in primary total hip arthroplasty. J Arthroplasty 2007;22(6 Suppl 2):140–4.
6. Griffin WL, Nanson CJ, Springer BD, et al. Reduced articular surface of one-piece cups: a cause of runaway wear and early failure. Clin Orthop Relat Res 2010;468(9):2328–32.
7. Squire M, Griffin W, Mason J, et al. Acetabular component deformation with press-fit fixation. J Arthroplasty 2006;21(6 Suppl 2):72–7.
8. Davies A, Willert H, Campbell P, et al. An unusual lymphocytic perivascular infiltration in tissues around contemporary metal-on-metal joint replacements. J Bone Joint Surg Am 2005;87(1):18–27.
9. Jacobs JJ, Skipor AK, Doorn PF, et al. Cobalt and chromium concentrations in patients with metal on metal total hip replacements. Clin Orthop Relat Res 1996;(Suppl 329):S256–63.
10. Pandit H, Glyn-Jones S, McLardy-Smith P, et al. Pseudotumours associated with metal-on-metal hip resurfacings. J Bone Joint Surg Br 2008;90(7): 847–51.
11. Willert H, Buchhorn G, Fayyazi A, et al. Metal-on-metal bearings and hypersensitivity in patients with artificial hip joints. A clinical and histomorphological study. J Bone Joint Surg Am 2005;87(1):28–36.
12. Amstutz H, Beaulé P, Dorey F, et al. Metal-on-metal hybrid surface arthroplasty—Surgical technique. J Bone Joint Surg Am 2006;88(Suppl 1 part 2): 234–49.
13. Langton D, Sprowson A, Mahadeva D, et al. Cup anteversion in hip resurfacing: validation of EBRA and the presentation of a simple clinical grading system. J Arthroplasty 2009;25(4):607–13.
14. Langton D, Jameson S, Joyce T, et al. A review of 585 serum metal ion results post hip resurfacing: cup design and position is critical. New Orleans (LA): American Academy of Orthopaedic Surgeons; 2010.
15. DeLee JG, Charnley J. Radiological demarcation of cemented sockets in total hip replacement. Clin Orthop Relat Res 1976;121:20–32.
16. Brooker A, Bowerman J, Robinson R, et al. Ectopic ossification following total hip replacement. Incidence and a method of classification. J Bone Joint Surg Am 1973;55(8):1629–32.
17. Kaplan E, Meier P. Nonparametric estimation from incomplete observations. J Am Stat Assoc 1958; 53:457–81.
18. Amstutz H, Su E, Le Duff M, et al. Are there benefits to one- versus two-stage procedures in bilateral hip resurfacing? Clin Orthop Relat Res 2010. [Epub ahead of print].
19. Della Valle C, Mesko N, Quigley L, et al. Primary total hip arthroplasty with a porous-coated acetabular component. A concise follow-up, at a minimum of twenty years, of previous reports. J Bone Joint Surg Am 2009;91(5):1130–5.
20. Engh C, Hopper RJ, Engh CJ. Long-term porous-coated cup survivorship using spikes, screws, and press-fitting for initial fixation. J Arthroplasty 2004; 19(7 Suppl 2):54–60.
21. Chiang P, Burke D, Freiberg A, et al. Osteolysis of the pelvis: evaluation and treatment. Clin Orthop Relat Res 2003;417:164–74.

22. Roth A, Winzer T, Sander K, et al. Press fit fixation of cementless cups: how much stability do we need indeed? Arch Orthop Trauma Surg 2010;126(2): 77–81.

23. Udomkiat P, Wan Z, Dorr L. Comparison of preoperative radiographs and intraoperative findings of fixation of hemispheric porous-coated sockets. J Bone Joint Surg Am 2001;83(4):1865–70.

24. Ball S, Le Duff M, Amstutz H. Early results of conversion of a failed femoral component in hip resurfacing arthroplasty. J Bone Joint Surg Am 2007; 89:735–41.

25. Schmalzried T. Metal-metal bearing surfaces in hip arthroplasty. Orthopedics 2009;32(9). Available at: http://www.orthosupersite.com/view.asp? rID=42831. Accessed January 19, 2011.

26. Mahendra G, Pandit H, Kliskey K, et al. Necrotic and inflammatory changes in metal-on-metal resurfacing hip arthroplasties. Acta Orthop 2009;80(6): 653–9.

27. Glyn-Jones S, Pandit H, Kwon Y, et al. Risk factors for inflammatory pseudotumour formation following hip resurfacing. J Bone Joint Surg Br 2009;91(12): 1566–74.

Sporting Activity After Hip Resurfacing: Changes Over Time

Michel J. Le Duff, MA, Harlan C. Amstutz, MD*

KEYWORDS

- Hip resurfacing • Sporting activity • Prosthesis
- Scoring • Hip arthroplasty

The evolution of patient sporting activities after hip resurfacing has not yet been studied. The Impact and Cycle Score (ICS), a scoring algorithm to quantify sporting activity, was developed to compare type of activity, frequency, duration, and overall activity level in the early postoperative period and at mid- to long-term follow-up. The scoring of the ICS included (1) the impact score (IS), which rated activities based on the predominant type of displacement involved and then multiplied this rating by frequency and duration scores, and (2) the hip cycle score (HCS), which rated activities based on the number of hip cycles per unit of time characterizing the activity and then multiplied this rating by frequency and duration scores. All patients were also evaluated using the University of California, Los Angeles (UCLA) hip scoring system. Mean time for the first survey was 1.8 years postoperatively (range, 1.0–4.9 years) and 9.1 years (range, 5.0–13.4 years) for the second survey.

Positive correlations were found between IS and the UCLA activity score and between HCS and the UCLA activity score. Mean IS decreased from 30.4 to 26.5 between the surveys ($P = .0116$), whereas the mean HCS decreased from 35.8 to 30.4 ($P = .0020$). Competitive participation increased from 5.5% to 10.1% among the listed activities ($P = .0129$), and high-impact sports increased from 12.4% to 17.5% among the listed activities ($P = .0454$). Patients younger than 50 years at

surgery maintained all activity scores between the surveys, whereas patients aged 50 or older showed a significant decline in IS, HCS, and UCLA hip score. Although the overall activity level remains high, especially in patients younger than 50 years at surgery, the older patients showed a decline in overall quantity of activity overtime. This decline could be a result of the natural aging process or a possible "wear off" effect of the initial enthusiasm for sporting activities associated with a successful hip procedure. However, the increase in competitive participation and the proportion of impact activities indicate the patients' confidence in the durability of the prosthesis.

Restoration of original lifestyle could be considered the ultimate goal of hip arthroplasty. Wright and colleagues[1] showed that returning to professional and recreational activities was the most important reason why patients undergo total hip arthroplasty (THA) aside from pain relief and improving walking function. These recreational activities often include sporting activities, especially in young patients for whom sports constitute an important part of overall physical activity.[2] It is now established that the patient population receiving metal-on-metal hip resurfacing devices is usually younger and more active than the general patient population receiving a conventional THA.[3–7]

Participation in sports after hip resurfacing has been described at short-term follow-up, with

Funding for this study was provided by Saint Vincent Medical Center, Los Angeles, and Wright Medical Technologies Inc.

Joint Replacement Institute at St Vincent Medical Center, The S. Mark Taper Building, 2200 West Third Street, Suite 400, Los Angeles, CA 90057, USA

* Corresponding author.

E-mail address: harlanamstutz@dochs.org

Orthop Clin N Am 42 (2011) 161–167

doi:10.1016/j.ocl.2010.12.001

orthopedic.theclinics.com

greater than 90% of the patients returning to sporting activities.[8-10] A randomized clinical trial found a difference in overall activity score in favor of hip resurfacing when compared with conventional THA.[11] High-impact activities were shown to have a detrimental effect on the survivorship of hip resurfacing with polyethylene bearings,[12] and surgeons usually agree that high-impact sports should not be recommended after a hip arthroplasty.[13,14] However, outcome of the procedure is likely affected by not only what patients do after surgery but also how much and how often. In addition, patient involvement in sports may not be constant over time, and no attempt has been made to study the evolution of the type, amount, and level of physical activity the patients regularly engage in after hip resurfacing.

The purpose of this study is to compare the nature of activities, frequency and intensity of participation, and duration of sessions between the short postoperative period and the mid- to long-term follow-up in a group of patients treated with metal-on-metal hip resurfacing arthroplasty.

MATERIALS AND METHODS
Instruments

Data collection was performed using a survey available online as an encrypted document. The patients were given the possibility to report up to three sporting activities that they were participating in on a regular basis. For each sport mentioned (chosen from an extensive list), the patient selected the frequency of participation and the duration of typical sessions. The intensity level was also recorded as patients were asked to indicate if they were participating competitively or for recreational purposes only. The patients also reported if they were beginner, intermediate, advanced, or expert level for each activity selected. The survey was filled out at each clinical follow-up with a minimum of 1 year postsurgery. UCLA scores[15] were recorded and SF-12 quality of life scores[16,17] were computed at the last follow-up. A scoring algorithm was developed to quantify the answers to the survey and named the *Impact and Cycle Score* (ICS).

The ICS included two scores:

1. Impact score (IS): activities were rated based on the predominant type of displacement involved and then multiplied by frequency and duration scores:
   Patient IS = Σ (Activity IS x F x D), where Activity IS is the impact score associated with an activity, F is the frequency score, and D is the duration score

2. Hip cycle score (HCS): activities were rated based on the number of hip cycles per unit of time characterizing the activity and then multiplied by frequency and duration scores:
   Patient HCS = Σ (Activity HCS x F x D), where Activity HCS is the hip cycle score associated with an activity, F is the frequency score, and D is the duration score.

Details of the scoring algorithm are presented in **Tables 1** and **2**.

For the IS scores, activities with no or minimal displacement were rated 1; activities for which walking was the primary mode of locomotion, or in which the hip joint reaction forces were limited (low impact) were rated 2; activities with limited displacement but some impact were rated 3; and activities for which the primary modes of displacement were running or jumping were rated 4.

For the HCS score, the activities were rated from 1 to 4 based on pilot data collected with pedometers or accelerometers to determine the number of hip cycles necessary per unit of time for each activity.

Subjects

Between 1996 and 2003, 547 patients (636 hips) received metal-on-metal surface arthroplasties and were asked to fill out the sports activity survey at least 1 year postsurgery and then yearly. Of these patients, 445 completed at least one survey between 1 and 5 years after surgery, and 201 of these filled out at least one subsequent survey 5 years or more after the initial data collection; these patients constituted the study group. The average age of the patients was 49.6 years (range, 15–77 years) and men accounted for 74.6% of the study group. The average weight was 82.7 kg (range, 47–164 kg) and average body mass index was 26.9 (range, 19–46). Initial causes included osteoarthritis (68%), developmental dysplasia of the hip (11%), osteonecrosis (8%), trauma (6%), and others (7%), including Legg-Calve-Perthes disease, slipped capital femoral epiphysis, epiphyseal dysplasia, rheumatoid disease, and pigmented villonodular synovitis. Of the patients who underwent hip surgery, 6% had undergone previous surgeries; 28% of the patients had bilateral hip resurfacing and 4% had various types of conventional THAs on the contralateral hip. Among the study group, 8 patients had undergone revision surgery between the surveys.

Implants and Surgical Technique

The prosthesis used in the present study was the Conserve® Plus (Wright Medical Technology,

Table 1
Scoring of the activities in which patients engaged

Activity	Impact Score	Hip Cycle Score
Aerobics	3	3
Archery	1	1
Badminton	4	3
Ballet/ballroom dancing	2	2
Baseball/softball	4	2
Basketball	4	3
Bowling	2	1
Canoeing	1	1
Cross-country skiing	2	4
Cycling	2	4
Downhill skiing (groomed)	2	2
Downhill skiing (moguls)	4	2
Cardio machine (eg, step, elliptical)	2	3
European handball	4	3
Golf (using a cart)	1	1
Golf (walking between holes)	1	3
Handball	4	3
Hockey	4	2
Horseback riding	1	1
Ice skating	2	2
Martial arts	4	2
Motocross riding	3	1
Pilates	1	1
Racquetball	4	3
Rock climbing	1	1
Rollerblading	2	2
Rugby	4	3
Rowing	2	2
Running	4	4
Sailing	1	1
Scuba diving	2	2
Soccer	4	3
Squash	4	3
Surfing	2	1
Swimming	1	1
Tennis (doubles)	3	2
Tennis (singles)	4	3
Volleyball	4	2
Walking, hiking, backpacking	2	3
Water skiing	2	2
Weightlifting	2	1
Wrestling	4	2
Yoga	1	1

The impact score (IS) is based on the predominant type of displacement inherent to each activity. The hip cycle score (HCS) is based on the number of hip cycles per unit of time characteristic from each activity.

Table 2
Scoring of the frequency and duration of sessions

Frequency of Sessions (times per month)	Frequency Score	Duration of Sessions (min)	Duration Score
1–4	1	0–30	1
5–8	2	30–60	2
9–12	3	60–120	3
>12	4	>120	4

Inc, Arlington, TN, USA). The surgical technique used for implanting the devices was described in a previous report.[18]

Statistics

The Wilcoxon signed-rank test was used to assess differences between early and last follow-up IS and HCS. Chi-square analysis was performed to determine changes in the nature and intensity of the sports participation. Pearson correlation coefficients were calculated between sports survey scores (IS and HCS) and the other outcome scores (SF-12 and UCLA). Reliability of the two ICS components was assessed through computation of intraclass correlation coefficients on a subset of 37 patients on whom data was collected twice within 1 month, with a minimum of 1 day between the two surveys.

RESULTS

Mean follow-up was 1.8 years (range, 1.0–4.9 years) for the first survey and 9.1 years (range, 5.0–13.4 years) for the second survey. At last follow-up, the mean UCLA hip scores of the study group were 9.5, 9.6, 9.5, and 7.7 for pain, walking, function, and activity, respectively. No differences were seen in UCLA activity scores recorded at the first and second surveys (7.8 vs 7.7, respectively; $P = .6769$). The SF-12 scores were 52.2 for the physical component and 54.3 for the mental component.

The number of patients participating in at least one sporting activity decreased from 193 (96%) in the initial survey to 180 (90%) at last follow-up ($P = .5003$). The number of activities listed by the patients decreased from a grand total of 498 (mean, 2.47 per patient) to 428 (mean, 2.13 per patient) ($P = .0214$). The most popular activities at the first follow-up point were walking, including hiking or backpacking (25.5%); cycling (16.9%); weightlifting (13.1%); swimming (9.0%); and golf

(9.0%). Overall, these popular low-impact activities represented 73.5% of the activities listed by the patients. At last follow-up, these five activities were still the most popular and represented 67.1% of the listed activities. This difference was not significant (*P* = .2448). High-impact activities (impact score of 3 or 4) represented 12.4% of the activities listed in the first survey. These increased to 17.5% of the listed activities at last follow-up (*P* = .0454).

At the first survey, competitive participation was associated with 5.5% of the activities, whereas at last follow-up, it represented 10.1% (*P* = .0129). In the initial survey, 33.9% of the patients engaged in their favorite activities more than 12 times per month, and at last follow-up, 33.3% had the same high frequency of participation. The spread of frequency in participation did not change between the surveys (*P* = .8866). The typical duration of the

sessions was 30 to 60 minutes (45% of the answers in the initial survey and 36% at last follow up), and no change was seen in the distribution of durations (*P* = .1483). Patients reported an advanced or expert level in 35.1% of their answers in the initial survey and in 36.5% of their answers at last follow-up. No difference (*P* = .7913) was seen between the surveys in how the patients viewed their own participation level (beginner, intermediate, advanced, or expert level).

The 37-patient test–retest reliability assessment yielded high intraclass correlation coefficients for the two components of the ICS, with 0.87 and 0.80 for IS and HCS, respectively. The mean IS was 30.4 (range, 0–128) at the first survey and 26.5 (range, 0–120) at the last follow-up (*P* = .0116). Similarly, the mean HCS was 35.8 (range, 0–144) at the first survey and 30.4 (range, 0–132) at the last follow-up (*P* = .0020) (**Fig. 1**).

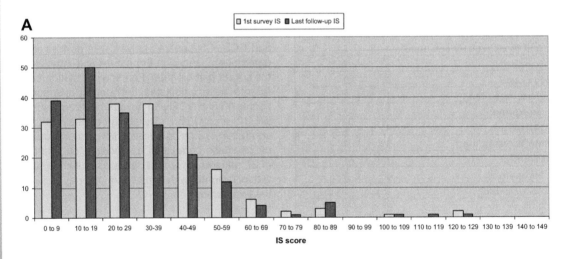

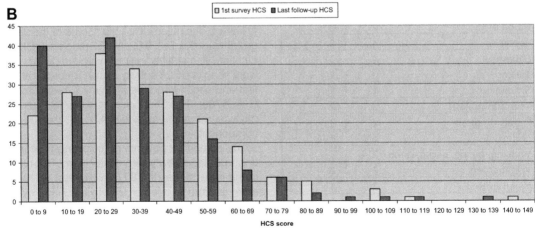

Fig. 1. (*A*) Distribution of impact scores (IS) from the initial survey and at last follow-up. The decline in IS between the surveys is shown by the larger number of scores between 0 and 20 at the time of the second survey. (*B*) Distribution of hip cycle scores (HCS) from the initial survey and at last follow-up. The decline in HCS between the surveys is shown by the larger number of scores between 0 and 30 at second survey.

A positive correlation was found between the UCLA hip score and both IS (r = 0.589; P<.001) and HCS (r = 0.564; P<.001). Both IS and HCS were also weakly correlated with the physical component of the SF-12 survey (r = 0.230; P<.05 and r = 0.267; P<.01, respectively). No association was found between IS or HCS and any of the other clinical scores (UCLA pain, walking, and function, and mental component of the SF-12). Also, no correlation was found among age at surgery and IS, HCS, and the UCLA activity score for the first or second survey (r = −0.12–0.16; P>.05). However, patients younger than 50 years (mean, 42.2 years) maintained both IS (29.7 vs 28.5; P = .5775) and HCS (34.2 vs 31.8, P = .366) over time, whereas the patients aged 50 years or older (mean, 57.2 years) showed a marked reduction in both IS (31.2 vs 24.5; P = .0033) and HCS (37.5 vs 28.9; P = .0003), as shown in **Fig. 2**. A similar result was found with the UCLA activity score, with patients younger than 50 years having an average score of 7.8 at first survey and 8.0 at second survey (P = .660), whereas the score among patients aged 50 years and older declined from 7.8 to 7.5 (P = .044).

In the group of eight patients (seven women and one man; mean age, 39.5 years) who had undergone revision surgery, the second survey was taken at an average of 65 months (range, 37–87) after the date of revision. The average IS was 35.0 (range, 2–80) for the first survey and 20.8 (range, 0–48) for the second survey (P = .116). The average HCS for the first survey was 32.0 (range, 3–68) and 26.6 (range, 0–60) for the second survey (P = .4222).

DISCUSSION

This study had the goal of describing and quantifying the sporting activity level of patients at short and mid- to long-term follow-up after hip resurfacing. One limitation of this study is that it was based on voluntary participation to fill out the survey, and therefore the study group only included 37% of eligible patients. However, the mean UCLA (in particular the activity score that has been identified as the best activity scale for patients undergoing joint arthroplasty[19]) and SF-12 scores were comparable to those previously published for the entire series,[20] and therefore the study group was a representative sample of the overall series.

This study shows that the participation of patients who underwent hip resurfacing in sporting activities is high and remains high at mid- to long-term follow-up. The rate of participation corroborates the findings of Banerjee and colleagues[8] or Naal and colleagues[9] at 2-years follow-up, or Narvani and colleagues[10] at 6 months' minimum follow-up.

Both the impact score and the hip cycle scores decreased significantly over time, which may be a result of the normal aging process or a possible "wear off" effect of the initial enthusiasm for sporting activities associated with a successful hip procedure. Because the frequency of participation and the duration per session remained the same between the two follow-up intervals, this decrease in overall scores can only be attributed to the lower number of activities the patients engaged in at last follow-up. The patients seemed to select preferential activities and abandoned the others over time. The most popular activities remained the same over time, with a clear preference of the patients for low-impact sports, suggesting a general adherence to the surgeon's recommendations. This finding is consistent with those of Naal and colleagues,[9] who showed that participation in high-impact sports decreased after surgery.

In contrast, this study noted a slight increase in participation to high-impact activities over time, which is somewhat surprising. A possible interpretation is that the patients gained confidence in the durability of the prosthesis and their own ability to resume these activities between the survey intervals. Greater confidence in skills and the reconstruction would also explain the higher percentage of participations listed as competitive versus recreational, which justifies the selection of preferential activities.

This study did not find any association between age at surgery and the level of activity (UCLA activity score, IS, or HCS), as suggested by Naal and colleagues.[9] However, the patients younger than 50 years who underwent surgery maintained their sporting activity levels between the surveys, whereas those who underwent surgery at age 50 years or older showed a marked decline also observed in the comparison of UCLA scores. This result is important because the population of patients who typically undergo surgery with hip resurfacing is very young, and the durability of the procedure will be affected by high activity levels for a much longer time than among the typical population of patients who undergo conventional THA. In addition, this result shows the importance of following up on patients' activity levels over time to determine any relationship with prosthetic durability.

The group of patients who underwent revision surgery between the surveys showed a trend toward a reduction of the IS (P = .116), but this did not reach significance, most likely because

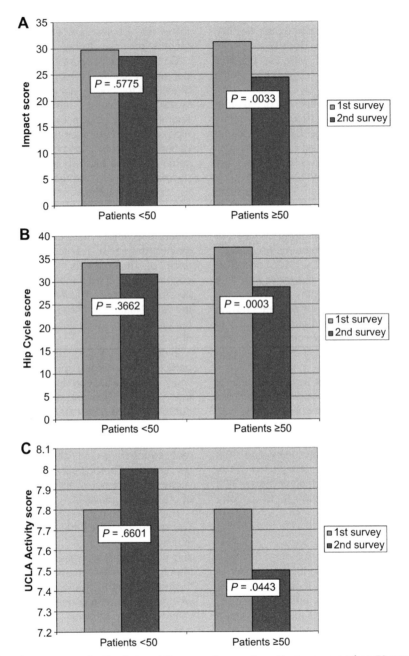

Fig. 2. (*A*) Mean impact scores for the first and the second survey in patients younger than 50 years and patients aged 50 years or older at surgery. (*B*) Mean hip cycle scores for the first and the second survey in patients younger than 50 years and patients aged 50 years or older at surgery. (*C*) Mean UCLA hip scores for the first and the second survey in patients younger than 50 years and patients aged 50 years or older at surgery.

the comparison of scores for only eight patients was underpowered.

The survey used in this study and its scoring algorithm provide much more information about patients' sporting activities than do already-established activity scores commonly used in the orthopedic community, and the authors

encourage other centers to collect data on the nature, but also the frequency and duration, of the patient's participation in sports. A parallel use of direct quantification of the number of hip cycles through pedometers or accelerometers could greatly complement a patient-based data collection such as the survey used in the present study.

However, performing these studies on large patient populations is logistically difficult and raises the issue of population sampling.

The quantification of sporting activity is a challenging undertaking but should become a useful tool in studying the relationship between failure rates and use of the prosthesis. Further follow-up may reveal the benefits or negative effects of certain activities on the durability of the reconstruction.

REFERENCES

1. Wright JG, Rudicel S, Feinstein AR. Ask patients what they want. Evaluation of individual complaints before total hip replacement. J Bone Joint Surg Br 1994;76(2):229–34.
2. Sequeira M, Rickenbach M, Wietlishbach V, et al. Physical activity assessment using a pedometer and its comparison with a questionnaire in a large population survey. Am J Epidemiol 1995;142(9):989–99.
3. Back D, Dalziel R, Young D, et al. Early results of primary Birmingham hip resurfacings. An independent prospective study of the first 230 hips. J Bone Joint Surg Br 2005;87(3):324–9.
4. Daniel J, Pynsent PB, McMinn D. Metal-on-metal resurfacing of the hip in patients under the age of 55 years with osteoarthritis. J Bone Joint Surg Br 2004;86(2):177–88.
5. De Smet K. Belgium experience with metal-on-metal surface arthroplasty. Orthop Clin North Am 2005;36(2):203–13.
6. Siebel T, Maubach S, Morlock M. Lessons learned from early clinical experience and results of 300 ASR hip resurfacing implantations. Proc Inst Mech Eng H 2006;220(2):345–53.
7. Treacy R, McBryde C, Pynsent P. Birmingham resurfacing arthroplasty. A minimum follow-up of five years. J Bone Joint Surg Br 2005;87(2):167–70.
8. Banerjee M, Bouillon B, Banerjee C, et al. Sports activity after total hip resurfacing. Am J Sports Med 2010;38(6):1229–36.
9. Naal F, Maffiuletti N, Munzinger U, et al. Sports after hip resurfacing arthroplasty. Am J Sports Med 2007;35(5):705–11.
10. Narvani A, Tsiridis E, Nwaboku H, et al. Sporting activity following Birmingham hip resurfacing. Int J Sports Med 2006;27(6):505–7.
11. Lavigne M, Masse V, Girard J, et al. Return to sport after hip resurfacing or total hip arthroplasty: a randomized study. Rev Chir Orthop Reparatrice Appar Mot 2008;94(4):361–7.
12. Kilgus DJ, Dorey FJ, Finerman GA, et al. Patient activity, sports participation, and impact loading on the durability of cemented total hip replacements. Clin Orthop Relat Res 1991;269:25–31.
13. McGrory BJ, Stuart MJ, Sim FH. Participation in sports after hip and knee arthroplasty: review of literature and survey of surgeon preferences. Mayo Clin Proc 1995;70(4):342–8.
14. Kuster M. Exercise recommendations after total joint replacement: a review of the current literature and proposal of scientifically based guidelines. Sports Med 2002;32(7):433–45.
15. Amstutz H, Thomas B, Jinnah R, et al. Treatment of primary osteoarthritis of the hip. A comparison of total joint and surface replacement arthroplasty. J Bone Joint Surg Am 1984;66(2):228–41.
16. Ware J, Kosinski M, Keller S. A 12-Item Short-Form Health Survey: construction of scales and preliminary tests of reliability and validity. Med Care 1996;34(3):220–33.
17. Ware J, Kosinski M, Keller S. SF-12: How to score the SF-12 physical and mental health summary scales. 3rd edition. Lincoln (RI): Quality Metric Inc; 1998.
18. Amstutz H, Beaulé P, Dorey F, et al. Metal-on-metal hybrid surface arthroplasty. Surgical technique. J Bone Joint Surg Am 2006;88(Suppl 1 Pt 2):234–49.
19. Naal F, Impellizzeri F, Leunig M. Which is the best activity rating scale for patients undergoing total joint arthroplasty? Clin Orthop Relat Res 2009;467:958–65.
20. Amstutz H, Le Duff M. Eleven years of experience with metal-on-metal hybrid hip resurfacing: a review of 1000 conserve plus. J Arthroplasty 2008;23(6 Suppl 1):36–43.

Reducing Metal Ion Release Following Hip Resurfacing Arthroplasty

David J. Langton, MRCS[a,b,c,]*, Thomas J. Joyce, PhD[c],
Navjeet Mangat, MRCS[a,d], James Lord, MEng[a,c],
Maarten Van Orsouw, MD[a,e], Koen A. De Smet, MD[a,e],
Antoni V.F. Nargol, FRCS (Tr & Orth)[a,b]

KEYWORDS

- Metal ion release • Resurfacing arthroplasty • Implant
- Ion concentration

Increased chromium (Cr) and cobalt (Co) concentrations following metal-on-metal (MoM) hip arthroplasty are associated with local and systemic pathologic changes.[1–6] It is unquestionable that efforts should be made to identify modifiable variables leading to ion release to minimize the risk of adverse effects.

To date, the variables that have been shown to significantly affect metal ion concentrations in the absence of renal disease are femoral component diameter,[7] acetabular cup angles of inclination and anteversion,[7–9] time from surgery,[10] and activity.[11] Of these variables, only cup orientation can be regarded as realistically under the surgeon's control. However, it remains to be proven whether an optimal cup position exists and whether this is affected by implant design. Our previous work and those of others have suggested that the coverage angle provided by the acetabular cup is critical.[7,12]

There is evidence, concordant with laboratory data, to suggest that clearance may also be an important variable in determining in vivo wear rates.[13]

There were 3 aims of this study:

1. To investigate the relationship between volumetric wear rate and serum metal ion concentrations
2. To establish the incidence of excessive metal ion release following resurfacing with commonly used devices
3. To identify cup orientations associated with lowest ion concentrations for each device and to propose mechanisms leading to increased wear.

PATIENTS AND METHODS

There were 723 patients in this series, 446 men and 277 women. All surgeries were performed by

Disclosure: David Langton has received payment for work as a consultant to DePuy and Wright Medical; Koen De Smet is a consultant for Wright Medical.
The remaining authors have nothing to disclose.
None of the authors/authors' families have any commercial or financial interest in the material in the study.
[a] Joint Replacement Unit, University Hospital of North Tees, Hardwick, Stockton-on-Tees, TS19 8PE, UK
[b] North Tees and Hartlepool NHS Trust, University Hospital of North Tees, Hardwick, Stockton-on-Tees, TS19 8PE, UK
[c] School of Mechanical and Systems Engineering, Newcastle University, Stephenson Building, Claremont Road, NE1 7RU, England, UK
[d] Northern Deanery, North East Strategic Health Authority, Waterfront 4, Goldcrest Way, Newburn Riverside, Newcastle Upon Tyne, NE15 8NY, UK
[e] ANCA Medical Centre, Krijgslaan 181, 9000, Ghent, Belgium
* Corresponding author. 199 Rodsley Avenue, Gateshead, NE8 4LB, UK.
E-mail address: djlangton22@doctors.org.uk

Orthop Clin N Am 42 (2011) 169–180
doi:10.1016/j.ocl.2011.01.006

2 experienced hip resurfacing surgeons who use metal ion analysis as part of routine follow-up. Both surgeons perform more than 100 hip resurfacings per year. Surgeon 1 is based in the United Kingdom (at site 1) and surgeon 2 is based in Belgium (at site 2). At both sites, blood samples were collected from the patients at a minimum time of 12 months after surgery to avoid the confounding factor of higher levels of wear during the run-in period.[14,15] These patients did not have any other metal implants at the time of measurement. Three resurfacing devices were studied: the Articular Surface Replacement (ASR; DePuy International, Leeds, UK), the Birmingham Hip Resurfacing (BHR; Smith and Nephew, Warwick, UK), and the Conserve® Plus (C+; Wright Medical Technology, Memphis, TN, USA). Serum ion analysis was performed using inductively coupled plasma mass spectrometry. Volumetric wear rates of explanted components determined by coordinate measuring machine analysis were compared with corresponding serum ion concentrations in vivo. The relationships between ion levels and component size and cup orientations remaining in vivo were investigated. The mean (range) age of patients from site 1 was 56 years (25–83 years) and the mean (range) time from surgery to blood sampling was 29 months (12–72 months) for the patients with the ASR implant device and 66 months (48–81 months) for those with the BHR implant device. The mean age of patients from site 2 was 51 years and the mean (range) time from surgery to blood sampling was 19 months (12–29 months) for the patients with the ASR implant device, 51 months (12–106 months) for those with the BHR implant device, and 28 months (12–54 months) for those with the C+ implant device.

Implants

From site 1, there were 223 patients with ASR and 72 with BHR implants. From site 2 there were 271 patients with BHR, 136 with C+, and 21 with ASR implants. **Table 1** shows the differences in design between the implants in this study.

Sample Collection

The samples were obtained at site 2 using an intravenous catheter (Insyte-WTM; Becton Dickinson, Franklin Lakes, NJ, USA). After the catheter had been introduced, the metal needle was withdrawn and the first 5 mL of blood was discarded to avoid possible contamination from the needle. A second 5 mL was collected using a vacuum tube (Venosafe VF-106SAHL; Terumo Europe NV, Leuven, Belgium). The samples were analyzed at the Laboratory of Clinical Biology at Ghent University Hospital, Ghent, Belgium. The laboratory quotes its quantification limit as 0.5 μg/L with a reproducibility of 5%. At site 1, serum samples were collected in a similar manner. Venous cannulation was performed with a 21-gauge stainless steel needle (Venflon, Becton Dickinson, Helsingborg, Sweden), with disposal of the first 5 mL of blood to avoid contamination. All samples were centrifuged to separate blood and serum fractions, frozen, and sent for blinded trace element analysis at the Trace Element Laboratory of the Royal Surrey County Hospital, Guildford, United Kingdom. This laboratory also quotes its quantification limit as 0.5 μg/L with a reproducibility of 5%.

Radiographic Analysis

At the time of collection of the sample, the University of California, Los Angeles activity scores were

Table 1
Comparison of device characteristics

Device Characteristics	ASR	BHR	C+
Subtended articular surface angle (°)	144–160[a]	158–165[a]	162–165[a]
Mean nominal radial clearance (μm)	50	100	80
Manufacturing method of head	As cast	As cast	HIP/SA[b]
Manufacturing method and treatment of cup	HIP/SA[b]	As cast	HIP/SA[b]
Carbon content[c]	High	High	High

[a] Subtended articular surface angles increase with increasing cup diameter.
[b] HIP/SA, cast process and heat treatment by hot isostatic pressure/surface annealed.
[c] High carbon content defined as ≥0.20%.
 Data from Heisel C, Kleinhans JA, Menge M, et al. Ten different hip resurfacing systems: biomechanical analysis of design and material properties. Int Orthop 2009;33(4):939–43; manufacturers' details; and independent testing.

recorded and weight-bearing pelvic radiographs were obtained. From these radiographs, the following parameters were measured using ImageJ software (National Institutes of Health, Bethesda, MD, USA): femoral stem angle relative to the femoral shaft (SSA), femoral stem to femoral neck angle (SNA), and femoral offset and femoral component to femoral neck ratios. Einzel-Bild-Roentgen-Analyse (EBRA, University of Innsbruck, Innsbruck, Austria) software was used to analyze all available radiographs to obtain angles of cup inclination and anteversion. The accuracy of this software has been discussed in the literature.[16] In most cases, one well-centered radiograph was available for analysis. Theoretical contact patch to rim (CPR) distance was calculated for all patients.[17]

To test the validity of comparing Cr and Co levels between the 2 populations, patients with BHR implants from site 2 were matched with patients with BHR implants from site 1 by the length of time to blood sampling from surgery. From these patients, we selected only those with femoral components of size 50 mm and larger as we have previously showed these sizes to be relatively resistant to cup position.[7,17] To further control for the effects of cup position, cups with inclinations greater than 55° and less than 10° or anteversion greater than 30° were excluded. The Cr and Co levels for the matched populations were then compared using Mann-Whitney tests for nonparametric data (**Table 2**). P values less than .05 were deemed significant. Two sample t-tests comparing the relevant parameters can be seen in **Table 2**. Cr concentrations in patients from UK were found to be slightly but significantly increased when compared with patients from Belgium. There was no significant difference between the groups with regard to Co. For this reason, we used only serum Co in the analysis.

For the 3 resurfacing devices, the relationship between each variable and serum Co was examined using the Spearman rank correlation. Rank correlation was preferred because of the nonparametric nature of the ion data. Scatter plots were used to identify nonlinear relationships. To examine the relative sensitivity of each device to the effects of cup orientation, the patients from each implant group were divided into subgroups of inclination (<25°, 25°–27°, 27°–29°, 29°–31°, 31°–33°, 33°–35°) and anteversion (<0°, 0°–5°, 5°–7°, 7°–9°, 9°–11°). From each subgroup the median Co level was calculated and plotted. To further examine this relationship, patients were placed into zones of cup orientation based on the EBRA measurements (**Fig. 1**). We then calculated the percentage of patients in each zone (for each device) with serum Co levels more than 7 μg/L. This figure has recently been quoted by the Medicines and Healthcare Products Regulatory Agency/Metal on Metal Working Committee of the United Kingdom, indicating a poorly performing bearing surface with recommendations for close patient follow-up. Windows SPSS version 15.0 (SPSS Inc, Chicago, IL, USA) was used for statistical analysis throughout.

Survival Analysis Using Metal Ion Concentrations

In our previous work we showed that there was a suggestion that there is a temporary immunity to increases in the wear of malpositioned cups/cups.[17] With this principle in mind, we collected all the metal ion results from all patients in the study at all periods, including repeat samples from individual patients at different times postoperatively. Of the 723 patients, 124 had undergone repeat testing (as part of routine screening), giving a total of 847 samples. Using these data, we conducted a Kaplan-Meier survival analysis comparison between the patients in each device group, with the latest follow-up being the time in months

Table 2
Comparison of joint sizes/orientations and serum Cr and Co concentrations of patients with the BHR implant device from both sites

Variables	Site 1	Site 2	P value
Number	40	48	—
Time to Sample (mo)	66 (48–81)	64 (50–81)	.190
Femoral Size (mm)	51.6	52.4	.107
Cup Inclination (°)	48.5 (33–55)	48.8 (34–55)	.890
Cup Anteversion (°)	17.04 (10–39)	20.5 (10–36)	<.001
Serum Cr (μg/L)[a]	3.49	1.80	<.001
Serum Co (μg/L)[a]	1.31	1.20	.812

[a] Median values, all other values are means (range).

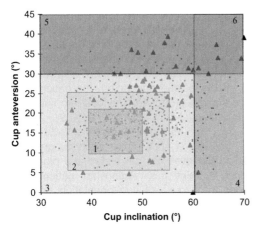

Fig. 1. Cup orientation zones. Serum Co concentrations in zone 1 were significantly lower than that in zones 2 to 6 (P = .04 zone 1 vs zone 2). Zones 2 and 3 represent gradual extension of zone 1. Zone 1: inclination, 40° to 50°; anteversion, 10° to 20°. Zone 2: inclination, 35° to 55°; anteversion, 5° to 25°. Zone 3: inclination, 30° to 60°; anteversion 0° to 30°. Zones 4 to 6 represent suboptimally orientated cups as previously defined by resurfacing metal ion studies.[7,12,17] Zone 4: inclination greater than 60°; anteversion less than 30°. Zone 5: inclination less than 60°; anteversion greater than 30°. Zone 6: inclination greater than 60°; anteversion greater than 30°.

from the resurfacing to the last blood sample. The patients were then categorized into a large joint group (femoral diameter≥53 mm) or a small joint group (femoral diameter<53 mm). The principle of this categorization was based on our previous results, which showed larger joints to be less vulnerable to the effects of cup position.[17] The patients were then also categorized by cup position and a Cox proportional hazard model constructed.

EXPLANT ANALYSIS

The wear of retrieved ASR matched femoral and acetabular components from site 1 (n = 35 pairs) was measured by a coordinate measuring machine (CMM) using a scanning head (Legex 322, Mitutoyo Halifax, UK) with a spatial resolution of less than 1 μm in the area of measurement. Measurements were made for every 5° on 18 concentric circles as well as at the pole of the component, which resulted in a total of 4500 to 6000 measurements for each component, dependent on the radius of the explant. The wear scars of each component were categorized as anteverted or retroverted according to the description by Walter and colleagues.[18] Volumetric wear was calculated using the method described in the Appendix. Univariate linear

regression was used to examine the relationship between volumetric wear rates and serum Co and Cr levels. Using the Medicines and Healthcare products Regulatory Agency (MHRA) level of 7 μg/L as a positive test and abnormal bearing surface wear as an annual wear rate greater than 3 mm^3/y, (In our recent work, 3 mm^3/yr was the lowest bearing surface wear rate of a resurfacing device associated with adverse reaction to metal debris.[19]) the sensitivity and specificity of serum Cr and Co testing was evaluated.

RESULTS A: EX VIVO
Explant Analysis and Serum Ion Concentrations

Volumetric wear correlated well with serum Cr (r^2 = 0.66, P<.01) and serum Co concentrations (r^2 = 0.78, P<.01). Specificity and sensitivity (95% CI) of serum Co levels greater than 7 μg/L were found to be 1.00 (0.67–1.00) and 0.93 (0.83–0.98), respectively. Specificity and sensitivity (95% CI) of serum Cr levels greater than 7 μg/L were found to be 0.80 (0.48–0.97) and 0.93 (0.83–0.97), respectively. Wear maps of retrieved components were generated and can be seen adjacent to the corresponding radiographs (**Fig. 2**). In **Fig. 2**, for simplification, red areas represent wear of greater than 20 μm deviation from a perfect spherical form. All explants that were found to have extremely high wear rates were found to have edge loading of the acetabular components. We define edge loading here as a progressive increase in the measured wear depths of the cups so that maximal wear depths occur at the edge of the articular surface.

RESULTS B: IN VIVO
Femoral Size

In all 3 devices, we identified an inverse relationship between femoral component size and serum Co concentrations (**Table 3**). This relationship was not significant in the C+ device. However, the largest values were found in the patients in whom larger-diameter bearings had been suboptimally positioned.

Cup Inclination

Increasing serum Co concentrations were associated with increasing inclination angle of the ASR cup (**Fig. 3**; see **Table 3**). In the patients with BHR and C+ implant devices, lowest ion levels were associated with cups placed with inclinations of 45° to 50°. These results were consistent through the size ranges.

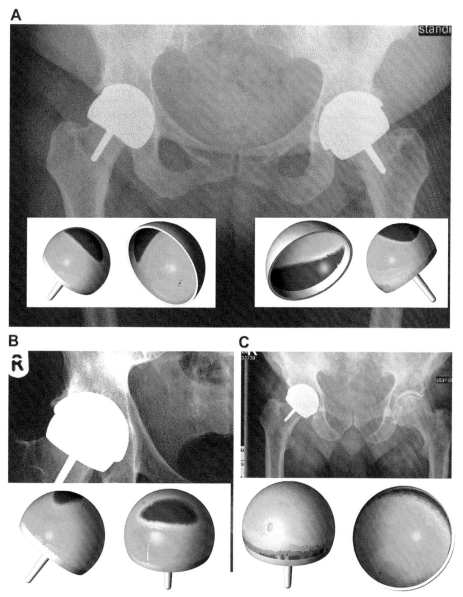

Fig. 2. (*A*) Retrieved components of a 45-year-old female patient with bilateral ASR resurfacings. Right ASR failed at 19 months, the left failed at 58 months. Both failures were secondary to pain, large joint effusions, and areas of tissue necrosis. The right cup was placed with inclination/anteversion angles of 57°/27°, and the corresponding femoral component shows signs of anterior rim loading with possible anterior subluxation. The left cup was placed with inclination/anteversion angles of 41°/0°. The wear scar is directed in an opposite direction to the right, indicating posterior rim loading and subluxation. The time to onset of pain in the left hip was much longer compared with the right and this potentially reflects the less steep increase in metal ion levels associated with low cup angles as opposed to high cup angles. (*B*) Femoral component of a 49-year-old male patient (ASR) with femoral fracture at 4 years associated with metallosis/aseptic lymphocyte dominated vasculitis associated lesion. The main wear scar is retroverted suggesting that the mechanism of wear was posterior edge loading/subluxation during deep flexion and internal rotation. The cup is orientated in 40° of inclination and 8° of anteversion (radiological). (*C*) Retrieved components from a 50 year old male who suffered a femoral neck fracture at 7 months. The cup was placed in 41° of inclination and 20° of anteversion. Patterns of wear suggest possible equatorial bearing secondary to low clearance.

Table 3
The Spearman rank correlations between each examined variable and serum Co concentration for each device

Variables	ASR	BHR	C+
Femoral Size	−0.22 (.01)	−0.21 (<.01)	−0.12 (.16)
Cup Inclination	0.41 (<.01)	0.09 (.07)	−0.11 (.20)
Cup Anteversion	0.15 (.130)	0.13 (.03)	0.20 (.021)
Time from Surgery	0.17 (.05)	0.07 (.50)	−0.07 (.432)
SSA	0.06 (.53)	0.18 (.05)	0.18 (.03)
SNA	−0.07 (.57)	0.18 (.190)	0.01 (.90)
Stem Neck	−0.14 (.17)	0.04 (.457)	0.25 (.05)
Offset	0.01 (.98)	−0.23 (.004)	−0.01 (.93)
UCLA Score	−0.29 (.09)	0.010 (.85)	−0.05 (.54)
Head Neck Ratio	0.47 (.01)	0.22 (<.01)	0.12 (.17)
CPR	−0.49 (<.01)	−0.255 (<.01)	−0.09 (.28)
Age	0.02 (.82)	0.06 (.65)	0.10 (.25)

All patients in the study are included. Note that there is a strong positive correlation among the patient group as a whole between femoral size and offset/SSA/SNA. When femoral size is controlled for these variables nonsignificant relationships to Co levels is shown. *P* values are given in parentheses.
Abbreviations: SSA, femoral stem angle relative to the femoral shaft, SNA, femoral stem to femoral neck angle.

Cup Anteversion

The ASR proved to be extremely sensitive to both increased and decreased anteversion (**Fig. 4**). The median Co concentration of patients with BHR devices with cups placed with anteversion greater than 30° was greatly increased, although this relationship was absent in patients with BHR devices with femoral implant sizes larger than 50 mm. The C+ device proved to be relatively resistant to the effects of anteversion; however, there were only a limited number of patients (n = 4) with a cup anteversion greater than 30°.

The Interaction of Bearing Diameter and Cup Orientation

Large joints of each device were compared with small joints of each device in cup zone 3, 4, and 5. These zones were selected because cups placed in these positions are not generally viewed as optimally placed, but they are commonly encountered

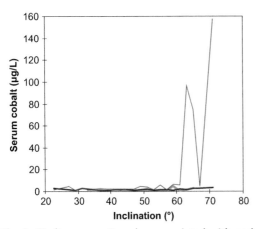

Fig. 3. Median serum Co values associated with each subgroup of inclination. All patients in the study are included. Red, ASR patients; blue, BHR patients; green, C+ patients. Median Co level associated with ASR cup inclinations greater than 60° is removed for graphical representation (21.5 µg/L).

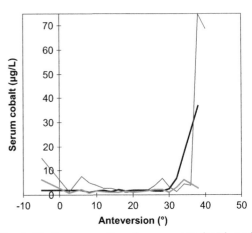

Fig. 4. Median serum Co values associated with each subgroup of anteversion. All patients in the study are included. Red, ASR patients; blue, BHR patients; green, C+ patients.

in surgical practice. In all devices, the median Co values were found to be lower in the large joint groups, 3.71 versus 2.38 µg/L ($P = .08$) for the ASR, 2.50 versus 1.60 µg/L ($P<.01$) for the BHR, and 3.00 versus 1.35 µg/L ($P = .04$) for the C+ groups.

Design Factors Other than Bearing Diameter and Cup Orientation

Site 2 patients with the BHR device were matched with those with the C+ device according to the duration of time postoperation to blood sampling. These 2 devices were selected for comparison because they have the largest arcs of cover, opposing heat treatments and differing clearances (see **Table 1**). From these patients, we selected only those with femoral components of size 50 mm and above for reasons outlined earlier. To further control for the effects of cup position, cups with extreme inclinations ($>55°$) and/or anteversions ($<10°$ or $>30°$) were excluded. The Cr and Co levels for the matched populations were then compared using Mann-Whitney tests for nonparametric data. Two sample t-tests comparing the relevant parameters of the 2 groups can be seen in **Table 4**.

Incidence of Serum Co Levels Greater than 7 µg/L Between Devices by Cup Placement Zone

Fig. 5 shows the percentage of patients with serum Co concentrations greater than 7 µg/L related to the zone of cup placement. In zone 1, serum Co concentrations in 10% of the patients with the ASR device were above this level. The C+ device was most resistant to variations in cup placement, consistent with the results described earlier. However, blood samples in patients with the BHR device were taken at a significantly greater period

postoperatively compared with the patients with the C+ device, hence our reason to conduct the survival analysis described later.

RESULTS C: SURVIVAL ANALYSIS

Direct comparison of the 3 devices with all patients and all results included showed a significant increase in the failure rate of the ASR device compared with the BHR and C+ devices (**Fig. 6**). There was no significant difference in survival between the groups with C+ and BHR devices. When patients with the large-joint implants were examined separately, there were no significant differences in the survival of each device and cup orientation was not found to be a significant variable. When only patients with the small-joint implants were included in the Cox hazards model, the ASR device was found to have a hazard ratio of 7.58 compared with the BHR device ($P<.01$). There was a sequential increase in the hazard ratio with cups placed further from zone 1 (all P values $<.05$).

DISCUSSION

Serum metal ion concentrations have been shown to correlate well with maximum wear depths of explanted femoral resurfacing prostheses.[1] However, linear wear depths can be unrepresentative of total volumetric loss of material. In this study, we have demonstrated for the first time a strong correlation between serum ion concentrations and total volumetric wear rates. Recently, there has been a report of multiple end organ damage secondary to Co intoxication after a conventional total hip replacement.[6] It has also been shown that revision surgery secondary to adverse reactions to metal debris frequently lead to unsatisfactory outcomes due to widespread tissue destruction.[20,21] It could be argued that reducing articulating surface wear is the most

Table 4
Comparison of joint sizes/orientations and serum Cr and Co concentrations of the matched patients with BHR and C+ devices from site 2

Joint Characteristics	BHR	C+	P value
Number	21	35	—
Time to Sample (mo)	34 (12–57)	28 (12–54)	.207
Size (mm)	52.2	51.5	.240
Cup Inclination (°)	50.7 (41–55)	50.3 (33–55)	.771
Cup Anteversion (°)	16.8 (10–19)	16.0 (10–19)	.326
Serum Cr (µg/L)*	2.00	1.60	.13
Serum Co (µg/L)*	1.80	1.10	.02

Figures are means (and range) unless denoted by "*" which indicate median values.

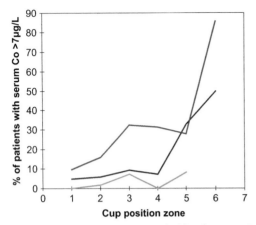

Fig. 5. Cup orientation zone and risk of serum Co concentrations greater than 7 μg/L. Red, ASR patients; blue, BHR patients; green, C+ patients.

important consideration when a resurfacing device is implanted, given the proven and theoretical risks of local and systemic exposure to metal debris. The Medicines and Healthcare Products Regulatory Agency of the United Kingdom have recommended close follow-up of patients with Co or Cr concentrations greater than 7 μg/L. The aim of this study was to gain further understanding of the risk of excessive metallic debris exposure after implantation of commonly used resurfacing devices by studying the largest independent metal ion collection in existence. We also hoped to provide evidence of the mechanisms leading to accelerated wear and suggest explanations as to why some devices and bearing sizes may be more susceptible to these processes.

Large diameter MoM joints are designed to harness a beneficial lubricating film to reduce wear. Components are manufactured with such precision that, in theory, the moving joint should develop a fluid film of sufficient thickness for the joint to function in fluid film lubrication (lambda ratio>3). It is recognized that harnessing of this lubricating film can be encouraged by increasing the femoral component size[22] and decreasing the clearance between the femoral and acetabular components.[13] Factors thought to impair fluid film generation include rim contact[23,24] and component subluxation.[25,26] If the prosthesis is starved of a lubricating film, wear will increase dramatically over the large bearing surfaces.[27] Evidence of this tendency to boundary lubrication in poorly performing prostheses can be found in the fact that the ion values considered statistical outliers in this data are found in the patients implanted with larger-diameter resurfacings.

Leslie and colleagues[26] showed in a hip simulator study that increased cup inclination angles (>55°) increased the rate of wear of resurfacing components secondary to edge loading. There is an expanding body of clinical data that is consistent with these results.[7–9] Leslie and colleagues also found that wear rates can be dramatically increased when edge loading is combined with microseparation of the femoral and acetabular components. This can best be achieved in clinical practice by combining high anteversion angles with high inclination angles. The joint is then vulnerable to posterior impingement of the femoral neck on the cup rim during extension, in some extreme cases during the gait cycle.[28] This mechanism in itself can disrupt the fluid film but can also lever the head anteriorly creating stripe wear on the femoral component and rim damage/edge wear on the cup (see **Fig. 2A**). In this way, the mechanical situation Leslie and colleagues showed to increase metallic wear 17-fold in vitro is potentially replicated in vivo.

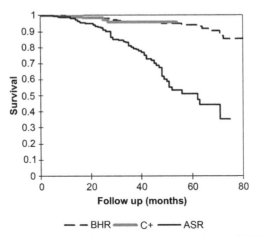

Fig. 6. Kaplan Meier survival analysis conducted using serum Co >7 μg/L as a failed joint.

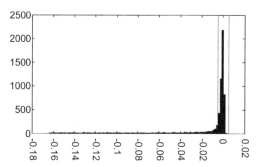

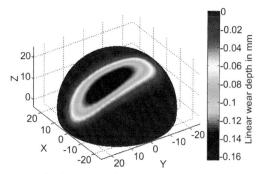

Fig. 7. A histogram showing the linear wear depths across the sample was created. Most points are very close to the zero mark, indicating that much of the surface was pristine. The vertical red lines represent +/− 5 microns around the determined radius. Most unused resurfacing devices we have examined have a manufactured form within this tolerance band.

Fig. 9. The heat map for the femoral head in **Fig. 8** colored by linear wear depth. Deep blue indicates maximum wear depth on the sample and deep red indicates a pristine surface.

The ASR device has a smaller arc of coverage relative to the other devices (see **Table 1**), which has certain implications. When matched for size and orientation, component contact always occurs closer to the rim of an ASR cup than in the other devices. The 3 cups, ASR, BHR, and C+, also have different rim designs. The ASR introducer inserts adjacent to the articular surface leaving a sharp edge, which may mean that subluxation of the ASR femoral component is particularly detrimental. The recessed nature of the articular rim in comparison with the outer rim also means that the advantage of a subhemispherical cup design in terms of avoiding impingement has been largely negated. It is to be noted that impingement is related to not only the cup design but also the angle of function of the femoral component. In practical terms, the ASR device does not provide a greater ROM than the other devices.

Healthy subjects require an average of 104° of hip flexion for sitting, 112° to rise from sitting, and 125° to stoop to pick up an object from the floor.[29] Hip extension reaches a mean peak of 20° during the normal adult gait cycle. Given this information, range of motion studies[30,31] involving hip resurfacing models suggest that the necks of resurfaced femurs frequently impinge on the acetabular cup during activities of daily living.[28] However, if impingement alone was the dominant mechanism of ion release, then wider variation is expected in the ion results associated with larger-diameter resurfacings because they have a poor head to neck ratio. This is clearly not the case. That is not to say that impingement is not an important factor, rather that the smaller variation in ion concentrations of larger diameter resurfacings are likely to reflect impingement processes without the compounding effect of severe edge loading. This theory may well explain why inclination angles of the C+ and BHR devices at the higher limit of what is presently considered acceptable (45°–50°) are associated with the lowest median ion levels in this large series. Inclination angles in this range, in these 2 devices, when coupled with reasonable angles of anteversion (10°–20°) confers a greater range of impingement-free flexion and extension as well as provides sufficient acetabular coverage.[30] The most recent anatomic studies of the human pelvis show the acetabular inclination angle to be approximately 55° (relative to the anterior pelvic plane).[32] It seems that once edge loading is eliminated as a factor, the more "physiologically" the acetabulum is reconstructed, the lower the associated metal ion concentrations.

Although there is clear evidence that the ASR cup favors lower inclination angles, there also seems to be a difference between devices in terms of the optimal angle of anteversion (see **Fig. 4**). The lowest median Co concentrations occur in

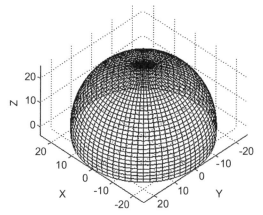

Fig. 8. An example of the grid created in Matlab for a femoral head.

Table 5
Comparison of the present method with established gravimetric methodology

Method	First	Second	Third
Gravimetric Weight (mg)	42.0	84.1	128.6
Gravimetric Volume (mm³)	5.1	10.1	15.5
Matlab: Mean ± Standard Deviation (mm³)	5.17 ± 0.72	9.82 ± 0.51	15.74 ± 0.25

patients with the ASR device with cups anteverted between 15° and 20°. In the group with the BHR device, lowest Co levels are found in patients with cups positioned between 10° and 15° of anteversion. The C+ seems to tolerate a wider range of anteversion. This tolerance leads us to speculate that the negative effects of near-neutral anteversion observed with the ASR and the smallest BHR devices are primarily because of the effects of posterior edge loading (±anterior impingement) during deep flexion/stair climbing. The retroverted wear scars identified on retrieved femoral components, which were coupled with cups with low angles of anteversion, provide direct evidence of this effect (see **Fig. 2**A, B).

We found a highly significant positive correlation between Co and Cr levels and head/neck ratio in the patients with ASR and BHR devices, that is, the greater the head to neck ratio, the higher the observed ion concentrations are likely to be. The head/neck ratio of the largest implants is approximately 1.30 steadily increasing up to 1.50 for the smallest implants (all devices). We consider this ratio to be further evidence that the radius and coverage arc of the bearing surface is more important than the head/neck ratio (ie, tendency to impinge) in the process of metal ion generation. We do not know if this is primarily because of an improved lubrication regime or because of the protection from edge loading. We must also not discount the possibility that a highly localized concentration of metal debris per se causes thinning of the femoral neck and consequently increases the head/neck ratio. However, analysis of serial radiographs does not seem to prove a clear association between neck thinning and metal ion levels at this stage.

Patients who have a well-positioned C+ device have a slightly but significantly lower Co concentration than those with a BHR device when the devices are comparable in terms of time to blood sampling, femoral size, and cup orientation. This may be because of the beneficial effect of or a combination of the reduced clearance of the C+, the larger acetabular coverage, and a difference in the material properties of the components. It does seem to suggest, however, that the heat treatment of the C+ device does not have a significant effect on ion release at this length of follow-up. This information must be taken with the caveat that the designer surgeon of the BHR (Derek McMinn) has shown evidence that a previous double heat-treated device first began to fail at 5 years postsurgery.[33] It was for this reason that we conducted our survival analysis.[33]

The survival analysis presented in this article must be interpreted with caution for obvious reasons. This study was not prospective and the time points at which blood samples were taken/repeated in each patient group were not standardized. Also, although blood tests at each center are performed routinely, significant selection bias cannot be ruled out. For example, patients experiencing pain may have been more likely to attend clinics to give samples. Despite this limitation, we believe that the large number of patients involved in the study go some way to reducing the effects of the factors described earlier. More importantly we do believe that the time from implantation to venesection plays a significant role in the identification of accelerated wear, particularly in poorly positioned or poorly designed implants. In the patient group described in this article, we identified 8 patients with ASR device with theoretical CPR distances of less than 5 mm who all had Co concentrations less than 7 μg/L in blood samples taken within 2 years of surgery. We have previously shown a CPR distance of less than 5 mm to be strongly associated with high wear states.[17] When these blood tests were repeated 2 years later, all but 2 of these patients were found to have Co levels greater than 7 μg/L. It is likely that this time delay is related to:

1. The duration of time that has to elapse before the edge of the developing wear area reaching the edge of the articular surface of the cup[24]
2. The time needed for the bearing surfaces to roughen beyond a critical level.

Either of these 2 situations could lead to the inability of the joint to develop a sufficient lubricating film and therefore an increased tendency toward boundary lubrication.[34]

Of the patients in this study, 13.6% were found to have serum Co concentrations greater than 7 μg/L. Increased concentrations were associated with reduced bearing diameter, suboptimal cup placement, and devices with reduced coverage arcs. In patients who received a BHR device or C+ resurfacing device with a femoral component larger than or equal to 49 mm mated with a cup placed between 30° and 60° of inclination and 0° and 30° of anteversion this percentage decreased to 3.35%.

Resurfacing cups positioned in 45° ± 5° of inclination and 15° ± 5° of anteversion seemed to be least vulnerable to the processes leading to metal ion release (see **Fig. 6**). Larger-diameter near-hemispherical components provide greater coverage and can tolerate greater variability in component orientation.

SUMMARY

The results of this study were consistent with the idea that the coverage arc provided by the resurfacing cup is critical in terms of metal ion generation. Smaller diameter bearings with insufficient coverage arcs are vulnerable to unacceptable increases in metal ion concentrations even when relatively well positioned. Of all the patients with the ASR device in this study, 23% were found to have Co concentrations greater than the MHRA guidance of 7 μg/L compared with 6% of the patients with the BHR and C+ devices. This incidence was further reduced to 3.4% when only patients with bearing diameters greater than or equal to 50 mm were included. Serum ion concentrations can reliably be used as surrogate markers of volumetric bearing surface wear.

APPENDIX

Cartesian coordinate data from the CMM were read into Matlab (The Mathworks, Inc, Natick, MA, USA). These data were used to reconstruct the surface of the component. At each point, the radius was calculated using the formula $\sqrt{X^2 + Y^2 + Z^2} = r$, where X, Y, and Z represent the Cartesian coordinates of the point and r is the radius of the sphere. By considering only the unworn regions of the samples, it was possible to identify the original component radius in this manner. It was important to disregard the worn areas in this stage because they would adversely affect the calculation. Using a histogram such as that in **Fig. 7**, it is obvious that the worn radii are the low frequency values and the unworn surface is represented by the high frequency values of small range. With the original radius known, the

linear wear depths were calculated by subtracting each calculated radius from the original radius. In the case of femoral heads, wear leads to a smaller radius being calculated. For acetabular cups, the calculated radii are larger.

Once the wear depths were calculated, a grid was interpolated between adjacent points (**Fig. 8**). This grid was used to calculate wear volume. The size of each grid square was calculated, and this size was multiplied by the mean wear depth at that square to give a volume. These small volumes were summed across the entire surface. A heat map was produced to show this information, allowing for quick visual analysis of wear severity and patterns (**Fig. 9**).

This method was validated against a gravimetric technique. A sample head was cleaned thoroughly in an acetone bath for 5 minutes. The sample head was left to dry for 1 hour on a lint-free cloth and then weighed on a high-precision scale (Denver Instrument, NY, USA, accuracy 0.1 mg). The sample was weighed 6 times and an average taken. After this, the sample was placed on the CMM using the method described earlier and the resulting data file was analyzed in Matlab. The sample then had a quantity of material removed to simulate wear and was cleaned, weighed, measured, and analyzed again in the same way. This procedure was repeated for a total of 4 times. The results are shown in **Table 5**.

REFERENCES

1. De Smet K, De Haan R, Calistri C, et al. Metal ion measurement as a diagnostic tool to identify problems with metal-on-metal hip resurfacing. J Bone Joint Surg Am 2008;90:202–8.
2. Hart AJ, Hester T, Sinclair K, et al. The association between metal ions from hip resurfacing and reduced T-cell counts. J Bone Joint Surg Br 2006;88:449–54.
3. Hart AJ, Skinner JA, Winship P, et al. Circulating levels of cobalt and chromium from metal-on-metal hip replacement are associated with CD8+ T-cell lymphopenia. J Bone Joint Surg Br 2009;91(6):835–42.
4. Hart AJ, Sabah S, Henckel J, et al. The painful metal-on-metal hip resurfacing. J Bone Joint Surg Br 2009;91(6):738–44.
5. Counsell A, Heasley R, Arumilli B, et al. A groin mass caused by metal particle debris after hip resurfacing. Acta Orthop Belg 2008;74(6):870–4.
6. Oldenburg M, Wegner R, Baur X. Severe cobalt intoxication due to prosthesis wear in repeated total hip arthroplasty. J Arthroplasty 2009;24(5):825, e15–20.
7. Langton DJ, Jameson SS, Joyce TJ, et al. The effect of component size and orientation on the concentrations of metal ions after resurfacing arthroplasty of the hip. J Bone Joint Surg Br 2008;90:1143–51.

8. Brodner W, Bitzan P, Meisinger V, et al. Serum cobalt levels after metal-on-metal total hip arthroplasty. J Bone Joint Surg Am 2003;85:2168–73.

9. Vendittoli PA, Mottard S, Roy AG, et al. Chromium and cobalt ion release following the Durom high carbon content, forged metal-on-metal surface replacement of the hip. J Bone Joint Surg Br 2007;89:441–8.

10. Daniel J, Ziaee H, Pradhan C, et al. Six-year results of a prospective study of metal ion levels in young patients with metal-on-metal hip resurfacings. J Bone Joint Surg Br 2009;91:176–9.

11. Khan M, Kuiper JH, Richardson JB. The exercise-related rise in plasma cobalt levels after metal-on-metal hip resurfacing arthroplasty. J Bone Joint Surg Br 2008;90:1152–7.

12. De Haan RD, Pattyn C, Gill HS, et al. Correlation between inclination of the acetabular component and metal ion levels in metal-on-metal hip resurfacing replacement. J Bone Joint Surg Br 2008;90:1291–7.

13. Rieker CB, Schön R, Konrad R, et al. Influence of the clearance on in-vitro tribology of large diameter metal-on-metal articulations pertaining to resurfacing hip implants. Orthop Clin North Am 2005;36(2):135–42.

14. Heisel C, Streich N, Krachler M, et al. Characterization of the running-in period in total hip resurfacing arthroplasty: an in vivo and in vitro metal ion analysis. J Bone Joint Surg Am 2008;90(Suppl 3):125–34.

15. Back D, Young DA, Shimmin AJ. How do serum cobalt levels change after metal-on-metal hip resurfacing? Clin Orthop 2005;438:177–81.

16. Langton DJ, Sprowson AP, Mahadeva D, et al. Cup anteversion post hip resurfacing arthroplasty: validation of EBRA and presentation of a simple clinical grading system. J Arthroplasty 2010;25(4):607–13.

17. Langton DJ, Sprowson AP, Joyce TJ, et al. Blood metal ion concentrations after hip resurfacing arthroplasty: a comparative study of articular surface replacement and Birmingham Hip Resurfacing arthroplasties. J Bone Joint Surg Br 2009;91:1287–95.

18. Walter WL, Insley GM, Walter WK, et al. Edge loading in third generation alumina ceramic-on-ceramic bearings. J Arthroplasty 2004;19:402–13.

19. Langton DJ, Joyce TJ, Jameson SS, et al. Adverse reaction to metal debris following hip resurfacing: the influence of component type, orientation and volumetric wear. J Bone Joint Surg Br 2011;93(2):164–71.

20. De Haan R, Campbell PA, Su EP, et al. Revision of metal-on-metal resurfacing arthroplasty of the hip: the influence of malpositioning of the components. J Bone Joint Surg Br 2008;90:1158–63.

21. Grammatopolous G, Pandit H, Kwon YM, et al. Hip resurfacings revised for inflammatory pseudotumour have a poor outcome. J Bone Joint Surg Br 2009;91:1019–24.

22. Smith SL, Dowson D, Goldsmith AA. The effect of femoral head diameter upon lubrication and wear of metal-on-metal total hip replacements. Proc Inst Mech Eng H 2001;215:161–70.

23. Morlock MM, Bishop N, Zustin J, et al. Modes of implant failure after hip resurfacing: morphological and wear analysis of 267 retrieval specimens. J Bone Joint Surg Am 2008;90:89–95.

24. Tuke MA, Scott G, Roques A, et al. Design considerations and life prediction of metal-on-metal bearings: the effect of clearance. J Bone Joint Surg Am 2008;90:134–41.

25. Bowsher JG, Nevelos J, Williams PA, et al. Severe wear challenge to as-cast and double heat-treated large-diameter metal-on-metal hip bearings. Proc Inst Mech Eng H 2006;220:135–43.

26. Leslie I, Williams S, Isaac G, et al. High cup angle and microseparation increase the wear of hip surface replacements. Clin Orthop Relat Res 2009; 467:2259–65.

27. Charnley J. Low friction arthroplasty of the hip. Heidelberg-New York. Berlin: Springer Verlag; 1981.

28. Ball ST, Schmalzried TP. Posterior femoroacetabular impingement (PFAI) after hip resurfacing arthroplasty. Bull Hosp Joint Dis 2009;67(2):173–6.

29. Amstutz H, Lodwig R, Schurman D, et al. Range of motion studies for total hip replacements. A comparative study with a new experimental apparatus. Clin Orthop 1975;111:124.

30. Williams D, Royle M, Norton M. Metal-on-metal hip resurfacing the effect of cup position and component size on range of motion to impingement. J Arthroplasty 2009;24(1):144–51.

31. Kluess D, Zietz C, Lindner T, et al. Limited range of motion of hip resurfacing arthroplasty due to unfavorable ratio of prosthetic head size and femoral neck diameter. Acta Orthop 2008;79(6):748–54.

32. Murtha PE, Hafez MA, Jaramaz B, et al. Variations in acetabular anatomy with reference to total hip replacement. J Bone Joint Surg Br 2008;90:308–13.

33. Daniel J, Ziaee H, Kamali A, et al. Ten-year results of a double-heat-treated metal-on-metal hip resurfacing. J Bone Joint Surg Br 2010;92-B:20–7.

34. Joyce TJ, Langton D, Jameson SS, et al. Tribological analysis of failed resurfacing hip prostheses and comparison with clinical data. Proc IME J J Eng Tribol 2009;223:605–6.

Incidence and Significance of Femoral Neck Narrowing in the First 500 Conserve® Plus Series of Hip Resurfacing Cases: A Clinical and Histologic Study

Karren M. Takamura, BA[a], James Yoon, BA[a],
Edward Ebramzadeh, PhD[b], Patricia A. Campbell, PhD[b],
Harlan C. Amstutz, MD[a],*

KEYWORDS

• Hip resurfacing • Metal-on-metal • Clinical outcomes
• Neck narrowing

Metal-on-metal hip resurfacing is an attractive option for young patients, as it leaves more femoral bone stock if revision surgery is necessary. It also restores normal anatomy and biomechanics of the hip, while providing near-normal proximal femoral anatomy and loading.[1] Narrowing or thinning of the femoral neck after metal-on-metal hip resurfacing arthroplasty has been reported as a common radiologic feature.[2–4] Although the long-term effects of neck narrowing are unknown, it has been speculated that neck narrowing does not result in adverse clinical or radiologic outcomes.[2]

This study reports the incidence and significance of neck narrowing in the first 500 consecutive hips in the senior surgeon's (H.C.A.) series with a relatively long follow-up and determines the cause where possible. The radiological features of neck narrowing were examined over time, as well as the clinical features and histology of retrievals of those hips that failed with neck narrowing.

MATERIALS AND METHODS

Between 1996 and 2002, the senior author (H.C.A.) implanted the first 500 consecutive Conserve® Plus metal-on-metal hip resurfacings (Wright Medical Technology, Inc, Arlington, TN, USA) in 431 patients (319 men, 112 women). The mean

One author (P.C.) has received research support from Wright Medical Technologies, Inc.
The institution of the authors (H.C.A., K.M.T.) has received funding from Wright Medical Technologies Inc and the St Vincent Medical Center Foundation.
[a] Joint Replacement Institute, St Vincent Medical Center, 2200 West Third Street, Suite 400, Los Angeles, CA 90057, USA
[b] University of California Los Angeles/J. Vernon Luck Orthopaedic Research Center, 2400 South Flower Street, Los Angeles, CA, USA
* Corresponding author.
E-mail address: harlanamstutz@dochs.org

Orthop Clin N Am 42 (2011) 181–193
doi:10.1016/j.ocl.2011.01.002

age at the time of surgery was 48.6 years, and the average follow-up was 95.9 (range, 1.4–161) months. Two patients were lost to follow-up. Neck narrowing was measured using a modified protocol used by Hing and colleagues.[2] Immediate postoperative radiographs were compared with the most recent postoperative radiographs for narrowing of the femoral neck at the component-neck junction (**Fig. 1**). All radiographs used were standardized anteroposterior (AP) views. Nonsuitable radiographs were excluded from the measurement (eg, femoral orientation not consistent with the rest of the series). Radiographic measurements of acetabular abduction and anteversion were made using the EBRA program (Einzel-Bild-Roentgen-Analysis, University of Innsbruck, Austria), and this program was also used to outline the femoral ball to find the center of the femoral head. Using the outline and the center of the femoral head, the Image J software (National Institute of Health, version 1.41) was used to measure the femoral ball diameter and the diameter of the neck at the component-neck junction. This procedure was performed by 2 independent observers (J.Y., K.M.T.). Radiographs that showed narrowing were evaluated at different time points over the series of follow-up visits to track changes in narrowing. The neck narrowing measurements were plotted against time to examine the progression of narrowing over the follow-up period. The

femoral head diameter was used to calibrate the radiographs to measure the amount of neck narrowing in millimeters and to calculate the percentage of narrowing. Cases exceeding 10% narrowing were further classified depending on whether the narrowing involved most of the neck or was caused by the presence of a more localized triangular area or "bite," with loss of bone at the component-neck junction and sclerotic line at the bite (**Fig. 2, Table 1**). Furthermore, the narrowing was assessed as either symmetric (both inferior and superior narrowing) or eccentric (mostly inferior or mostly superior narrowing). This assessment was done by the senior author (H.C.A.).

After the initial analysis of neck narrowing, we performed a secondary biomechanical analysis similar to that of Joseph and colleagues[5] to measure the abductor moment arm (AMA) and body moment arm (BMA) in 301 preoperative and 478 postoperative radiographs to calculate the hip ratio (HR), which indicates the force exerted by the abductor muscles and body weight to maintain equilibrium in the 1-leg stance (**Fig. 3**).[6] In addition, the stem shaft angle (SSA) was calculated for each hip. Radiographs without the entire AP view of the pelvis or with incomplete view of the greater trochanter were excluded from the biomechanical analysis. For the preoperative biomechanical analysis, 279 radiographs were available for the non–neck narrowing group and 22 for the neck narrowing group. For the postoperative biomechanical analysis, 446 radiographs were available for the non–neck narrowing group and 25 were available for the neck narrowing group.

The difference in preoperative and postoperative HR was calculated to assess changes in hip biomechanics. Clinical and radiologic variables including the underlying diagnosis, biomechanical and radiographic parameters (neck narrowing, abduction, anteversion, contact-patch-to-rim [CPR] distance as described by Langton and colleagues,[7] SSA, preoperative and postoperative HR, change in HR, postoperative AMA, postoperative BMA), demographic data (age, height, weight, body mass index [BMI], femoral head size), and patient assessment scores (Harris hip score [HHS], University of California Los Angeles [UCLA] activity score) were compared between the neck narrowing and non–neck narrowing groups.

Two-tailed Student *t*-tests were used to compare parametric data. Mann-Whitney-U tests were used to compare nonparametric data. A *P* value of less than 0.05 was deemed to be significant. χ^2 Analysis with Fisher exact test correction was used to compare the ratio of failure with nonfailure cases

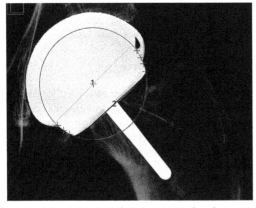

Fig. 1. Measurements taken to assess the degree of neck narrowing. A modified measurement previously described by Hing and colleagues[2] was used. Instead of measuring the diameter of the component at the component-neck junction, we measured the diameter of the actual femoral ball because it was a known measurement that can be used to calibrate the radiographs. Then the ratio of the femoral diameter (1) to the neck diameter at the component-neck junction (2) was compared with those on radiographs taken at further follow-up.

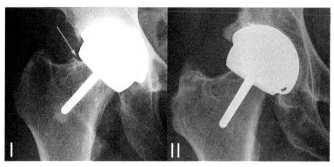

Fig. 2. The 2 general types of narrowing that were observed in our study. Hips in category I showed characteristic bite at the component-neck junction (*arrow*), an acute narrowing. Hips in category II showed a more uniform narrowing down the femoral neck shaft.

between the groups with and without neck narrowing.

Retrieved implants were examined at the Implant Retrieval Laboratory at the Los Angeles Orthopaedic Hospital. Upon retrieval, the specimens were fixed in formalin. The retrieved implants were subsequently cleaned, photographed, and examined grossly. Then the femoral component and associated femoral neck were sectioned using an EXAKT saw (EXAKT Advanced Technologies, Norderstedt, Germany) into 2.5-mm slices, which were then radiographed. These slices were removed from the metal, decalcified, and processed into paraffin for routine histologic examination and staining by hematoxylin-eosin. The cut sections that included the femoral neck, neck implant junction, and resurfaced bone portions were examined for osteoclastic and osteoblastic activity, as well as viability of the bone, which was assessed by the presence of nuclei in the bone. Soft tissues adhering to the neck and interfacial membranes were examined for the presence of inflammatory cells and wear debris.

RESULTS

Twenty-five hips in 22 patients were identified in the first 500 hips to have neck narrowing greater than 10%, which gives an incidence of 5%. In hips with neck narrowing, there were 11 males (13 hips, 52%) and 11 females (12 hips, 48%). In

hips without neck narrowing, there were 311 males (358 hips, 77.2%) and 106 females (117 hips, 25.2%). There was a significant difference in gender between the two groups (Chi-squared, $P = .001$), with a higher proportion of females in the neck narrowing group, occurring in 3.6% of male hips and 10.3% female hips.

There was no difference in the underlying diagnosis among cases with neck narrowing compared with the rest of the cohort (χ^2, $P = .36$) (**Table 2**). There was 20.1% (10.8%–38.7%) narrowing in the neck narrowing group, and the narrowing measured 7.1 mm (3.5–14.2 mm) at the last follow-up (mean, 101 months).

There were no differences in the age, weight, BMI, SSA, HHS, or UCLA activity score (**Table 3**). Height and femoral component size were significantly smaller in the neck narrowing group compared with the non–neck narrowing group only in men ($P = .0001$ and $P = .02$, respectively).

There were no significant differences in acetabular abduction, anteversion, or SSA (**Table 4**). The neck narrowing group had a significantly lower CPR ($P = .04$) and postoperative BMA ($P = .02$). There were no significant differences in the postoperative AMA and HR.

Six hips were classified into the first category, with the bite occurring at the component-neck junction (**Fig. 4**, **Table 5**). Case 1 was an 18-year-old patient with severe femoral cystic degeneration secondary to Legg-Calvé Perthes disease; the component was seated on the superior neck and implanted with a cemented stem. The hip recently loosened on the acetabular side after 10 years and is now pending revision (**Fig. 5**). Case 4 had an area of osteopenia superiorly and developed a bite at the component-neck junction, which did not progress during the past 4 years. The patient is active and plays racquetball (UCLA activity score 10) (**Fig. 6**). Case 5 had severe bone stock deficiency with large defects

Table 1	
Neck narrowing classification	
Category	Description
I	Neck narrowing with a bite at the component-neck junction
II	Neck narrowing involving most of the neck

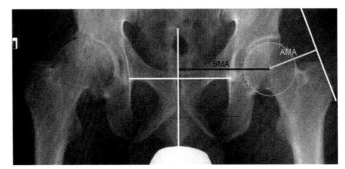

Fig. 3. Biomechanical measurements made in our study, the same measurements that were made in a study by Joseph and colleagues.[5] BMA and AMA measurements were made to calculate the HR.

and osteopenia inferiorly. The bite also occurred inferiorly; however, the narrowing is mostly taking place superiorly. Although narrowing is progressive, the patient is doing well at 10 years (**Fig. 7**).

Eighteen hips were classified into the second category, in which the narrowing involved most of the neck, not just an acute narrowing close to the component-neck junction (**Fig. 8**). Although most have stabilized, there is 1 case that continued to narrow until it failed from femoral loosening (case 11) and 1 that continues to narrow (case 21) and may require revision for fluid-filled adverse local tissue reaction (ALTR) (**Fig. 9**). Cases 22 and 23

(a 40-year-old male patient) had bilateral osteonecrosis and failed coring and considerable femoral bone loss at surgery. The necks narrowed progressively but stabilized by 5 years, with no further progression. The right hip demonstrates condensation of the medial cortical bone and is doing well at 12.5 years postoperation (UCLA pain, walking, and function scores of 10, activity score of 6).

All 7 failures in the neck narrowing group occurred in category II, and revision has been recommended for 2 hips with fluid-filled ALTRs. The 7 revised hips in the neck narrowing group were in category II, 5 of which were symmetric, 1 of which

Table 2
Etiology

Etiology	No Neck Narrowing	Neck Narrowing	Total
OA	300 (63.2%)	15 (60%)	315 (63%)
ON	39 (8.2%)	2 (8%)	41 (8.2%)
DDH	55 (11.6%)	2 (8%)	57 (11.4%)
Posttrauma	38 (8%)	1 (4%)	39 (7.8%)
Inflammatory			
Inflammatory OA	9 (1.9%)	—	9 (1.8%)
Ankylosing Spondylitis	3 (0.6%)	1 (4.0%)	4 (0.8%)
JRA	3 (0.6%)	—	3 (0.6%)
RA	4 (0.8%)	—	4 (0.8%)
RD	1 (0.2%)	—	1 (0.2%)
Childhood disorders			
LCP	12 (2.5%)	1 (4%)	13 (2.6%)
SCFE	7 (1.5%)	2 (8%)	9 (1.8%)
Other			
Melorheostosis	1 (0.2%)	—	1 (0.2%)
Epiphyseal Dysplasia	3 (0.6%)	1 (4%)	4 (0.8%)
Total	475	25	500

Abbreviations; DDH, developmental hip dysplasia; JRA, juvenile rheumatoid arthritis; LCP, legg–calvá–perthes; OA, osteoarthritis; ON, osteonecrosis; RA, rheumatoid arthritis; RD, rhuematoid disease; SCFE, slipped capital femoral epiphysis.

Table 3
Clinical parameters

	No Neck Narrowing (n = 475)	Neck Narrowing (n = 25)	P Value
Age	49 (15.3–78.1)	46 (18.2–68.1)	.19
Height (cm) (male)	178.8 (158–198)	171 (157–183)	.0001
Height (cm) (female)	164.4 (140–183)	164.3 (155–178)	.92
Weight (kg) (male)	89.1 (57–164)	82.5 (57–99)	.24
Weight (kg) (female)	67.8 (42–107)	66.3 (50–103)	.70
BMI (kg/m^2) (male)	27.8 (18.4–46.4)	28.1 (22.3–33.4)	.51
BMI (kg/m^2) (female)	25.0 (17.5–42.3)	24.5 (19.0–32.5)	.88
Female Femoral Head Size (mm)	42	42	.61
Male Femoral Head Size (mm)	48	46	.02
HHS	93 (40.9–100)	89 (52.9–99.9)	.08
UCLA activity	7.3 (3–10)	7.2 (4–10)	.51

was narrowed inferiorly, and 1 of which was not able to be determined as a result of the cup obstructing the inferior view of the component-neck junction. There were 2 revisions for acetabular loosening (after an average of 105.9 months), 1 for femoral neck fracture after 50 months, 1 for a fluid-filled ALTR and high metal ions after 120 months, and 3 for femoral loosening (after an average of 84.4 months). One woman had bilateral femoral neck narrowing, and both sides failed because of femoral loosening. Both sides had extensive femoral cystic degeneration preoperatively and were performed with first-generation technique using a small femoral size (both 38 mm); these hips were loose radiographically (lucent lines around the stem) before the neck narrowed symmetrically. The component then loosened further and tipped into the varus.

In hips without neck narrowing, there were 34 revisions: 1 for acetabular loosening, 1 for recurrent dislocation, 20 for femoral loosening, 5 for neck fractures, 1 for sepsis, 4 for osteolysis, 1 for component size mismatch, and 1 for socket loosening with intraoperative pelvic central fracture with unstable initial fixation. The incidence of failure was significantly higher in the neck narrowing group (Fisher exact, $P = .003$), and the difference in survivorship between the groups were significant (log-rank test, $P = .001$) (**Fig. 10**). The neck narrowing group had a lower survivorship rate of 86.7% at 7.7 years compared with 93.6% in the non–neck narrowing group.

Table 4
Radiographic parameters

	Non Neck Narrowing	Neck Narrowing	P Value
Abduction	43.4° (22°–71.5°)	45° (16.2°–65.7°)	.39
Anteversion	16.9° (2.4°–51.2°)	17.7° (3.0°–39.6°)	.98
CPR (mm)	14.7 (0.9–23.8)	13.8 (3.2–21.3)	.04
SSA	137° (110°–163°)	136° (125°–147°)	.59
Preoperative HR[a]	0.54 (0.31–0.99)	0.55 (0.40–0.68)	.91
Postoperative AMA (mm)[b]	51 (32–70)	49 (35–60)	.77
Postoperative BMA (mm)[b]	87 (64–102)	84 (72–91)	.02
Postoperative HR[b]	0.59 (0.35–0.79)	0.59 (0.46–0.73)	.20
Change in HR[a]	−0.05 (−0.56–0.45)	−0.04 (−0.25 to 0.12)	.64

[a] For preoperative biomechanical analysis, 279 radiographs were available for the non–neck narrowing group and 22 were available for the neck narrowing group.
[b] For postoperative biomechanical analysis, 446 radiographs were available for the non–neck narrowing group and all 25 were available for the neck narrowing group.

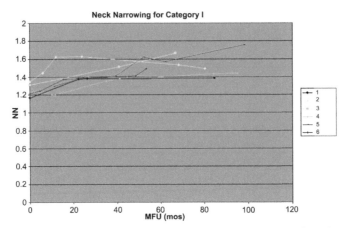

Fig. 4. The degree of neck narrowing (head diameter to neck diameter ratio) was plotted against time to look for signs of stabilization. These are the hips in category I.

There were 5 ALTRs in the neck narrowing group and 4 in the non–neck narrowing group (Fisher exact, P<.0001). Four of the ALTRs in the neck narrowing group were in category II and 1 hip for which the category was not determinable. Two of the ALTRs in the neck narrowing group were revised; 1 had a fist-sized solid mass, which was discovered incidentally at autopsy; and 2 have not been revised. The 2 unrevised cases are asymptomatic but are being monitored closely with metal ions and MRI. The femoral component in these patients averaged 44.4 mm. The average CPR distance was low, at 6.5 mm (3.2–9.8 mm), with the exception of 1 patient with a CPR distance of 21.3 mm because his cup was placed horizontally. At 10 years postoperation, 1 patient has an asymptomatic ALTR with high metal ions; although surgery was recommended, the patient has declined revision at this time and has received aspirations instead. All ALTRs in the neck narrowing group were fluid filled (n = 4), or in 1 case a solid mass, whereas all the ALTRs in the non–neck narrowing group were extremely active individuals who developed osteolysis in the neck and did not develop masses. All cases with osteolysis had small components (average, 41 mm) and underwent revision after an average of 98.4 months. Of 4 cases, 3 had satisfactory component orientation (average CPR, 11.7 mm). One case had malpositioning at 57.5° abduction and 34.3° anteversion (CPR, 4.2 mm), and this patient was very active, continuing her career in Tae Kwon Do. These osteolysis cases had high wear confirmed by coordinate measuring machine, CMM wear analysis.[8]

For the retrieval analysis, 2 failures (1 case of acetabular loosening, and 1 case of femoral neck fracture) were sectioned and examined histologically in the neck narrowing group.

The first patient was a 61-year-old woman who received a 44-mm Conserve® Plus resurfacing for osteoarthritis and underwent revision after 4 years for neck fracture. On sectioning the implant, it was clear that the component had a necrotic region that occupied the proximal portion of the femoral head adjacent to viable bone distally. The femoral neck had narrowed asymmetrically, and most of the narrowing took place inferiorly without a bite sign (category II-inferior). There was thick cortical bone inferiorly, and there seemed to be no active remodeling in this section. Distal bone appeared to be viable and to have consolidated, but without ongoing osteoblastic activity. There was no histologic evidence of abnormal osteoclastic activity in the area of radiographic narrowing.

Table 5
Radiographic characteristics and locations of neck narrowing

	Symmetric	Inferior	Superior	Total
Category I	1 (4.2%)	2 (8.3%)	3 (12.5%)	6 (25%)
Category II	14 (58.3%)	1 (4.2%)	3 (12.5%)	18 (75%)
Total	15 (62.5%)	3 (12.5%)	6 (25%)	24[a]

[a] One case of neck narrowing could not be determined because of excessive abduction and anteversion.

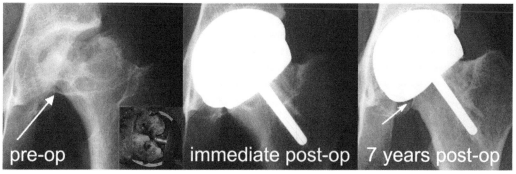

Fig. 5. An 18-year-old man with Legg-Calvé Perthes disease. The intraoperative photo shows severe cystic degeneration of the femoral head (*arrow*). At 7 years postoperation, there is a bite at the inferior femoral neck (*arrow*).

The second patient was a 57-year-old female dancer who received a 44-mm Conserve® Plus resurfacing for osteoarthritis. The acetabular component's initial orientation was 60° abduction and 23° anteversion and was obviously fibrous fixed with complete 3-zone socket radiolucency. However, the patient stayed active, teaching and performing ballet until the acetabular component migrated further and became painful at 117 months. The hip narrowed symmetrically (category II-symmetric) and progressively for 5 years before it stabilized, but it was difficult to measure when it migrated (**Fig. 11**). She underwent revision at 10 years because of acetabular loosening. The sectioned femoral component showed cortical thinning but without osteoclastic activity. The neck bone was lined by a fibrous membrane that was infiltrated with debris-filled macrophages. On the superior side below a cement-filled cyst, the bone trabeculae were thin and poorly interconnected but appeared to be viable.

DISCUSSION

The incidence of femoral neck narrowing greater than 10% reported in the hip resurfacing literature varies from 0% to 59% (**Table 6**). Our study found the incidence to be 5% in 500 hips with Converse Plus implants. Hing and colleagues[2] reported an incidence of 27.6% in a study of 163 Birmingham hip resurfacing (BHR, Smith and Nephew, Arlington, TN, USA) procedures (Smith and Nephew), which exceeded 10% narrowing at a mean follow-up of 5 years. Their study found neck narrowing to be associated with the anatomic neck-shaft angle (valgus femoral neck) and female gender, although statistical significance was only demonstrated for gender.

Past studies have shown narrowing to stabilize between 2 to 5 years[2,3,5] and suggest neck narrowing to be a relatively benign phenomenon. Although our study found that most cases stabilize, with a longer follow-up, some cases showed progressive narrowing and eventually failed; the

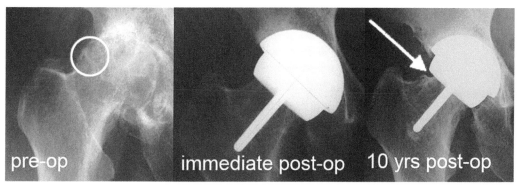

Fig. 6. Radiograph is of a 59-year-old woman with osteoarthritis implanted with a 42-mm component. The patient is extremely active, with a UCLA activity score of 10. Her hip is in category I, with the bite occurring superiorly (*arrow*); in the same area on her preoperative radiograph, there is an area of osteopenic bone (*circle*). The narrowing has stabilized after approximately 4 years.

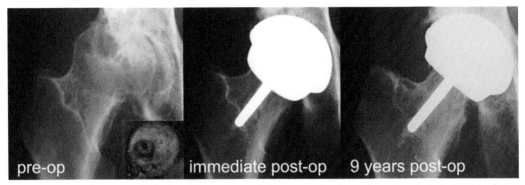

pre-op   immediate post-op   9 years post-op

Fig. 7. The bite can be seen inferiorly, whereas most of the narrowing has taken place inferiorly. The patient is doing well at 10 years postoperation.

number of failures was significantly higher in hips with neck narrowing. All of the published studies have a shorter study period, so it is possible that their studies were not long enough to detect any problems associated with neck narrowing.

Another notable comparison with other studies is our relatively low incidence of narrowing overall. This result may be attributed to a difference in the cementing technique and the 1-mm cement mantle for the hips in our studies. This technique allows for a uniform application of cement, which transfers stress more evenly to the neck periphery compared with the higher percentage in those systems without a cement mantle (eg, BHR, Cormet Corin), where liquid cement is applied from top down with lack of penetration of acrylic into the cylindrical portion. This procedure is in contrast to uncemented Cormet devices, in which stress shielding may contribute to what was observed as neck narrowing. Ho and colleagues[13] compared 54 cemented Cormet resurfacing devices with 33 uncemented devices and found the difference between the immediate

postoperative and last follow-up radiographs to be significant in patients with the cemented components but not the uncemented components. However, this study had a short follow-up period of 2 years.

Furthermore, these studies have not commented on the initial bone quality or cup positioning, which appears to play a role in neck narrowing. In our category I (bite) narrowing group, many cases had severe cystic degeneration or osteopenic bone in the areas of the neck that subsequently narrowed. If wear is associated with neck narrowing as hypothesized by Grammatopoulos and colleagues,[14] it is important that cup orientation is measured and CPR distance calculated to assess the risk of edge-loading and high wear.

Our study found significant differences in the height and component size in male patients with neck narrowing. Neck narrowing was associated with shorter men with smaller femoral components, which could explain why these patients also had significantly smaller CPR distances. Lilikakis and colleagues[11] also found that height

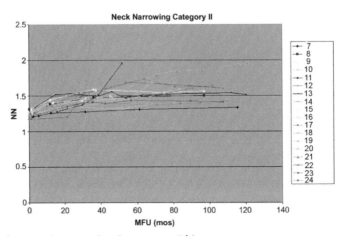

Fig. 8. Degree of neck narrowing over time in category II hips.

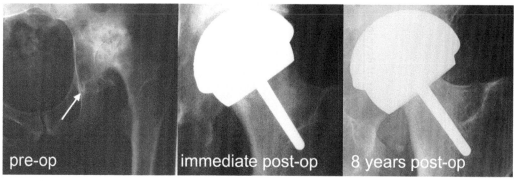

Fig. 9. In this case, the acetabulum was reconstructed above the anatomic location because of a severe pelvic fracture (*arrow*), and the socket was placed more horizontally. The narrowing is occurring both inferiorly and superiorly, and the radiograph at 8 years postoperation shows marked narrowing.

was significantly correlated with change in the cup to neck ratio; taller patients seemed to be more protected against neck thinning, and comparably, our study found patients with neck narrowing to be significantly shorter than patients without neck narrowing. Because there were no significant differences in component orientation, it is likely that the small component size contributed to the reduced CPR distance in the neck narrowing group.

Joseph and colleagues[5] found a correlation between the AMA and HR and femoral neck thinning in a study of 61 BHR procedures. Their study concluded that neck narrowing may be attributed to the altered biomechanics of the hip as a result of changes in the AMA and HR. Their study found

a significantly positive relationship between neck narrowing and AMA and AMA ratio, whereas they found a significantly negative relationship between neck narrowing and HR difference. Our study did not find a significant difference in HR or change in HR between hips with neck narrowing and hips without neck narrowing; the only significant difference we found was in the postoperative BMA. We were not able to compare differences in the preoperative and postoperative AMA and BMA because there was not a known distance to calibrate the measurements in the preoperative radiographs. The known femoral component size

Fig. 10. Difference in survivorship between hips with neck narrowing and hips without neck narrowing. Our study shows a longer follow-up observing this phenomenon compared with previously published studies. The neck narrowing group includes all hips in category I and II and 1 hip that was not categorized.

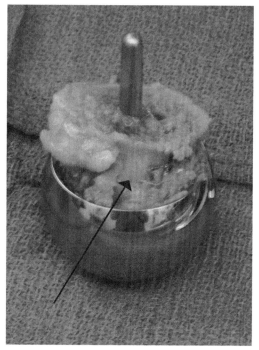

Fig. 11. The gross specimen retrieved at the revision surgery. The arrow shows the part of the femoral neck that has narrowed.

Table 6
This table summarizes the current studies that report the incidence of femoral neck narrowing and their follow-up period

Author	Journal	Year	Prosthesis	Follow-Up	Total Number of Hips Examined Radiographically	Hips with Neck Narrowing	Number of Revisions
Hing et al[2]	JBJS Br	2007	BHR	5 y (4–6)	163 hips	45 hips (27.6%), determined up to last follow-up	Not mentioned
Heilpern et al[9]	JBJS Br	2008	BHR	71 mo (60–93)	110 hips	16 hips (14.5%), determined up to last follow-up	4 hips
Jameson et al[10]	JBJS Br	2010	ASR	43 mo (30–57)	209 hips	124 hips (59.3%) determined at 2 y, with maximum 9% narrowing, no cases with narrowing >10%	12 hips
Joseph et al[5]	AOTS	2010	Cormet, BHR	3.6 y (2–5)	61 hips	39 (59%) determined at 2 y	0 hips
Lilikakis et al[11]	OCNA	2005	Cormet	28.5 mo (24–37.8)	63 hips	17 (27%) determined up to last follow-up	2 hips
Spencer et al[3]	TJA	2008	Corin Cormet	5.3 y (2–7)	40 hips	6 (15%) determined at 2 y, and tracked up to 7 y	2 hips
Steffen et al[12]	JBJS Br	2008	BHR	5.3 y (5–7.6)	85 hips	7 showed narrowing 6%–10%, no cases with narrowing >10% determined at review	23 hips of total 610 hips
Takamura et al (current study)	OCNA	2010	Conserve® Plus	8 y (0.1–13.4)	500 hips	25 (5%) determined up to last follow-up	41 hips

was used to calibrate the measurements in all of the postoperative radiographs.

However, we found a significantly higher prevalence of failure at 28% for hips identified with neck narrowing compared with 7.4% for hips without neck narrowing, observed up to a mean of 95.9 months. Although our results indicate a higher incidence of failure for the neck narrowing group, we agree with Joseph and colleagues[5] that an association between neck narrowing and femoral neck fracture is unlikely. Most fractures are short-term failures, and only 1 of 10 femoral neck fractures had neck narrowing greater than 10%, which was a long-term fracture.

In addition, our study found a significantly higher incidence of solid/fluid-filled mass-type ALTR in the neck narrowing group, in contrast to an osteolysis-type of ALTR associated with extremely high activity found in the non–neck narrowing group. Increased wear has been associated with the formation of ALTR[15] and neck narrowing, with metal particle–induced osteolysis and inflammation as possible contributing factors.[3,5] Grammatopoulos and colleagues[14] found that patients with inflammatory pseudotumors had a significantly higher head junction ratio, which signified narrower femoral necks, suggesting that pseudotumors may cause neck narrowing. Chen and colleagues[16] also found reactive masses in patients with neck narrowing, but their association with each other has not been proved. It is possible that an abnormal joint capsule environment, such as increased joint pressure resulting from these masses, could result in the narrowing of the neck because an osteolytic process was not identified on retrieval analysis.

Neck narrowing has been reported in patients without hip replacement prostheses. Goldberg and colleagues[17] reported 9 cases of femoral neck erosions in patients with pathologic processes in the hip joint. All 9 patients had abnormal synovial overgrowth or deposits as the underlying pathologic process. They observed that these erosions suggested a synovial process because the femoral head was often spared. Because the femoral neck is a bare area uncovered by the hyaline cartilage that covers the articulating surfaces, when synovial processes are severe enough to cause erosions, the femoral neck would be the first region to be affected. However, in our study, we did not encounter patients with synovial diseases in the neck narrowing group, although it is possible that other abnormal factors in the synovial joint could have led to femoral neck erosions.

We observed 2 distinct modes of narrowing in our series and categorized the cases accordingly. The interesting cases in the neck narrowing group were the hips with a bite at the component-neck junction. This bite feature has not been reported before, and it is possible that some of the previously reported cases of neck narrowing may in fact be a bite, which occurs at the component-neck junction, and a different process may be involved compared with the neck narrowing without these bites. It seems that in our study these bites are not associated with failure, as all the neck narrowing failures occurred in the group without the bite. All the hips in category I with the bites seemed to have bone quality issues that were found preoperatively in the same region. There were zones of osteopenia, severe bone defects, or large cysts, which may have contributed to the formation of these bitelike lesions in the postoperative period. Furthermore, there were 2 cases in which the impingement site was close to the component-neck junction, which may have contributed to remodeling at the component-neck junction, possibly contributing to bone loss at the component-neck junction (**Fig. 12**).

Our group previously studied a group of 18 hip resurfacing retrievals of different design types with neck narrowing[18] and found that regardless

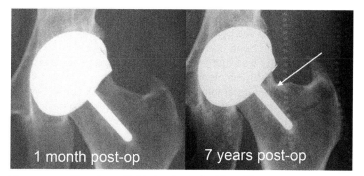

Fig. 12. A 78-year-old woman with osteoarthritis implanted with a 42-mm component. The patient developed a superior impingement sign (*arrow*). At the component-neck junction, neck narrowing is also apparent.

of reason for, or time to, revision, the neck histology showed similar features. The femoral heads that were studied were viable, and there were no cases of extensive avascular necrosis. Osteoclastic activity was notable in the femoral head in most cases, and it was often found in combination with new bone formation; thus, it seemed that the neck cortex appeared to be undergoing a process of reinforcement and re-modeling. In another study of 3 cases treated with cemented hemiresurfacing (but without a stem), the retrieval findings after an average of 17 years showed the original trabecular structure; extensive stress shielded bone loss was not seen, and no neck narrowing occurred.[19] However, in a study of 101 cemented stems versus nonce-mented stems in the same patients did not demonstrate any cases with neck narrowing.

The radiographic results described in our study represent what was measured only in the coronal plane. Neck narrowing in the sagittal plane was inconclusive, as there were an insufficient number of normalized lateral views suitable for examination. In addition, we were unable to standardize lateral views across nonnormalized radiographs and thus did not include these measurements in our study. Other studies have not measured neck narrowing in the sagittal plane for similar reasons.[3,5] Therefore, there is a possibility that the actual incidence of neck narrowing is greater than what we found or, in fact, may be circumfer-ential. Further study would be necessary with standardized lateral views to determine if changes in the neck are reflected by the coronal and sagittal planes equally or with computed tomography using artifact suppression techniques.

Even in the AP plane, there were some serial radiographs that were rotated, making the analysis impossible or difficult. Because of this rotation, there were limitations to the accuracy of our measurements. This problem can be seen in the graphs of the ratio of head to neck diameter versus time; it seems for some cases that the neck diam-eter is actually increasing. This increase was most likely because of the femoral component being slightly rotated or poor quality of the radiograph, where it is difficult to see where the bone cortex ends. Another limitation in our study was that we were not able to retrieve all failures for histologic analysis, which could have provided further infor-mation regarding the cause and histology of neck narrowing.

The multivariate model used by Lilikakis and colleagues[11] explained only 30% of the variance in change in the cup to neck ratio, suggesting the cause for neck narrowing to be multifacto-rial. Our study also confirms the multifactorial

nature of this process. We found height and component size to be a factor in men. A higher incidence of fluid or solid-mass ALTRs was found in the neck narrowing group, suggesting an association with increased wear in those cases. It is likely that neck narrowing can be attributed to different causes and many factors can contribute to this process, which is also evi-denced by the 2 distinct modes of narrowing that was found in our study.

Our study concludes that neck narrowing is associated with various factors, including female gender, shorter CPR distance, and shorter height and small component size in men. We have also found neck narrowing to be associated with a high-er incidence of failure and periprosthetic masses than the nonnarrowing group, in contrast to previous reports of neck narrowing being relatively benign. Because ALTR was not present in all cases of neck narrowing, it is unclear whether ALTR is a response to an abnormal synovial envi-ronment that also causes neck narrowing or if it is a primary contributor to the altered synovial envi-ronment. Therefore, it is important to follow-up patients with neck narrowing using metal artefact reduction sequence MRI to identify periprosthetic masses.

REFERENCES

1. Girard J, Lavigne M, Vendittoli P, et al. Resurfacing arthroplasty of the hip in osteopetrosis. J Bone Joint Surg Br 2006;88(6):818–21.
2. Hing C, Young D, Dalziel R, et al. Narrowing of the neck in resurfacing arthroplasty of the hip: a radio-logical study. J Bone Joint Surg Br 2007;89(8):1019–24.
3. Spencer S, Carter R, Murray H, et al. Femoral neck narrowing after metal-on-metal hip resurfacing. J Arthroplasty 2008;23:1105–9.
4. Ollivere B, Darrah C, Barker T, et al. Early clinical failure of the Birmingham metal-on-metal hip resur-facing is associated with metallosis and soft-tissue necrosis. J Bone Joint Surg Br 2009;91(8):1025–30.
5. Joseph J, Mullen M, McAuley A, et al. Femoral neck resorption following hybrid metal-on-metal hip resur-facing arthroplasty: a radiological and biomechan-ical analysis. Arch Orthop Trauma Surg 2010;130:1433–8.
6. Amstutz H, Beaulé P, Dorey F, et al. Metal-on-metal hybrid surface arthroplasty: two to six year follow-up. J Bone Joint Surg Am 2004;86:28–39.
7. Langton D, Sprowson A, Joyce T, et al. Blood metal ion concentrations after hip resurfacing arthroplasty: a comparative study of articular surface replace-ment and Birmingham hip resurfacing arthroplas-ties. J Bone Joint Surg Br 2009;91(10):1287–95.

8. Amstutz HC, Takamura, KM, et al. Wear analysis of 29 metal-on-metal hip resurfacing retrievals and relationship with "Adverse Local Tissue Reaction". 2011 Annual Meeting of the Orthopaedic Research Society. Long Beach (CA), 2011.

9. Heilpern G, Shah N, Fordyce M. Birmingham hip resurfacing arthroplasty: a series of 110 consecutive hips with a minimum five-year clinical and radiological follow-up. J Bone Joint Surg Br 2008;90(9): 1137–42.

10. Jameson S, Langton D, Nargol A. Articular surface replacement of the hip: a prospective single-surgeon series. J Bone Joint Surg Br 2010;92(1): 28–37.

11. Lilikakis A, Vowler S, Villar R. Hydroxyapatite-coated femoral implant in metal-on-metal resurfacing hip arthroplasty: minimum of two years follow-up. Orthop Clin North Am 2005;36(2):215–22.

12. Steffen R, Pandit H, Palan J, et al. The five-year results of the Birmingham hip resurfacing arthroplasty: an independent series. J Bone Joint Surg Br 2008;90(4):436–41.

13. Ho K, Beazley J, Parsons N, et al. Narrowing of the femoral neck after resurfacing arthroplasty of the hip: a comparison of cemented and uncemented femoral components. Hip Int 2010; 20(4):542–6.

14. Grammatopoulos G, Pandit H, McLardy-Smith P, et al. The relationship between head-neck ratio and pseudotumour formation in metal-on-metal resurfacing arthroplasty of the hip. J Bone Joint Surg Br 2010;92(11):1527–34.

15. Kwon Y, Glyn-Jones S, Simpson DJ, et al. Analysis of wear of retrieved metal-on-metal hip resurfacing implants revised due to pseudotumors. J Bone Joint Surg Br 2010;92:356–61.

16. Chen Z, Pandit H, Taylor A, et al. Metal-on-metal hip resurfacings-a radiological perspective. Eur Radiol 2010;21(3):485–91.

17. Goldberg R, Weissman B, Naimark A, et al. Femoral neck erosions: sign of hip joint synovial disease. AJR Am J Roentgenol 1983;141(1):107–11.

18. Campbell P, Takamura K, Shin B, et al. Histological features of femoral hip resurfacings with neck narrowing. The Annual Meeting of the Orthopaedic Research Society Meeting. New Orleans (LA), March 6–9, 2010.

19. Amstutz H, Esposito C, Campbell P. Long term preservation of femoral bone following hemiresurfacing. Hip Int 2010;20:236–41.

Imaging of Metal-on-Metal Hip Resurfacing

Catherine L. Hayter, MBBS[a], Hollis G. Potter, MD[b,c],*,
Edwin P. Su, MD[c,d]

KEYWORDS

- Hip resurfacing arthroplasty • Metal on metal
- Radiography • Magnetic resonance imaging
- Metal hypersensitivity • Osteolysis

Imaging of the painful surface replacement requires correlation between imaging and clinical data, including a comprehensive physical examination and careful patient history. The first mainstay of imaging evaluation is an appropriately performed radiograph to assess for radiographic findings that obviate more advanced imaging. In the setting of radiographs with equivocal or negative results, more advanced imaging may be necessary, and both magnetic resonance imaging (MRI) and ultrasonography have shown to be effective in the evaluation of these joints.[1–5] Ultrasonography is helpful in detecting periprosthetic fluid collections, which may then undergo ultrasound-guided percutaneous aspiration.[1,3,5,6] Computed tomography (CT) can detect osseous complications such as osteolysis[7] and allow more accurate assessment of component alignment.[2] Optimized MRI can not only identify fluid collections[2–4] but also assess for any adverse synovial response that may indicate wear-induced synovitis or infection as well as identify periprosthetic osteolysis.[8] Further modification of pulse sequences relevant to MRI is currently underway, resulting in marked improvement in the degree of artifacts generated by metal-on-metal (MOM) prostheses, allowing for superior characterization of the type of synovial reaction.

RADIOGRAPHIC ASSESSMENT

Because of its widespread availability, conventional radiography continues to be the primary imaging modality to evaluate the condition of hip resurfacing implants. With the ability to visualize a large field of view, conventional radiographs are able to assess implant position relative to the native anatomy of the hip, thus allowing the measurement of femoral stem-shaft and cup abduction angles. Sequential radiographs remain the preferred method of assessing implant stability over time, such as loosening. With proper radiographic technique, one can assess a hip resurfacing implant for position, heterotopic bone formation, periprosthetic lucency, impingement, osteolysis, migration, and neck narrowing.

Technique

Conventional radiographs should be taken in 2 planes to allow for biplanar evaluation of the

E.P.S. is a consultant of Smith and Nephew, Oklahoma City, OK, USA that provides research support.
Hospital for Special Surgery receives research support from General Electric Health Care.
The other authors have no conflicts of interest to disclose.

[a] Department of Radiology and Imaging, Hospital for Special Surgery, 535 East 70th Street, New York, NY 10021, USA
[b] Division of Magnetic Resonance Imaging, Department of Radiology and Imaging, Hospital for Special Surgery, 535 East 70th Street, New York, NY 10021, USA
[c] Department of Orthopaedic Surgery, Weill Medical College of Cornell University, 525 East 68th Street, New York, NY 10065, USA
[d] Department of Radiology and Imaging, Center for Hip Pain and Preservation, Hospital for Special Surgery, 535 East 70th Street, New York, NY 10021, USA
* Corresponding author. Division of Magnetic Resonance Imaging, Department of Radiology and Imaging, Hospital for Special Surgery, 535 East 70th Street, New York, NY 10021.
E-mail address: potterh@hss.edu

Orthop Clin N Am 42 (2011) 195–205
doi:10.1016/j.ocl.2010.12.006
0030-5898/11/$ – see front matter © 2011 Elsevier Inc. All rights reserved.

implant and surrounding bone. Most commonly, an anteroposterior view of the pelvis is taken in the frontal plane; visualization of both hips allows for a side-to-side comparison of the biomechanical axes of the hips. In the lateral plane, there is a wide variation in the preferred technique. At the authors' institution, the preferred view is the cross-table (shoot-through or Johnson[9]) lateral view. This radiograph is taken with the patient supine and the nonoperated hip flexed to 90° so that it does not obstruct the field of view. The beam is aimed from the midline, and the cassette is positioned lateral to the hip. This type of imaging allows visualization of the lateral plane of the cup position and assessment of the amount of anteversion and the presence of anterior cup overhang. Studies have debated the accuracy of the cross-table lateral view with regard to anteversion because of the variability in native pelvic tilt,[10] but this view still allows one to see the anterior aspect of the native acetabulum relative to the prosthetic edge (**Fig. 1**).

Interpretation

Femoral implant position

Conventional radiographs should be inspected for implant position. Commonly, the femoral stem-femoral shaft angle in both planes is of interest. This angle is assessed by measuring the angle created by a line drawn along the femoral stem and a line drawn down the femoral shaft (**Fig. 2**A). In the frontal plane, this angle typically approximates the native femoral neck-shaft angle of 135°, but several surgeons have advocated a more valgus orientation (higher stem-shaft angle) in order to improve the biomechanical forces on the neck.[11] In the lateral plane, the angle created by the femoral stem and femoral shaft should approximate the native version of the femoral neck; however, the angle may be directed from more posterior to anterior to improve bone contact

with the implant. Thus, there may be relative retroversion of the implant relative to the native femoral neck.

Acetabular implant position

Cup position is assessed by measuring the lateral edge of the acetabular component relative to a horizontal reference line in the frontal plane (see **Fig. 2**B). This abduction angle indicates the amount of lateral opening; typical values are 35° to 50°. Several studies have examined the effect of cup position on wear, and the steeper the cup angle (higher values) the greater the wear of an MOM implant.[12] Abduction angles greater than 55° are considered "steep," thus the preferred angle of an MOM surface arthroplasty is approximately 40° in the frontal plane.

In the lateral plane, anteversion of the socket is measured by the angle created from a vertical line perpendicular to the horizontal plane and the edge of the acetabular component (see **Fig. 2**C). Because of variation in technique, the true amount of anteversion may be obtained more accurately by Einzel-Bild-Roentgen-Analysis. Typical values for anteversion are similar to those of the native hip, measuring between 5° to 20°. Visualization of the anterior edge of the acetabular component is necessary to assess for protrusion of the component beyond the native bone, such as overhang of the component, which may lead to iliopsoas impingement and groin pain.

Implant stability

Sequential radiographs allow for the assessment of stability, over time, of an implant relative to bone. Implant migration, that is, change in position over time, is the sine qua non of a loose implant. Commonly, migration occurs on the femoral side and may be a result of osteonecrosis of the retained femoral head.

Most femoral resurfacing implants are cemented onto the retained femoral head and neck; the short

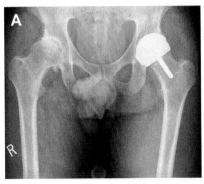
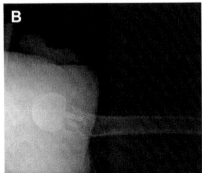

Fig. 1. Anteroposterior radiograph of the pelvis (*A*) and cross-table lateral radiograph of the left hip (*B*) demonstrates a left hip resurfacing implant.

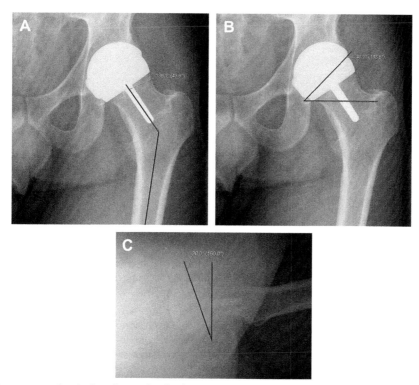

Fig. 2. (*A*) Anteroposterior (AP) radiograph of left hip resurfacing implant demonstrates measurement of the femoral stem-shaft angle, which typically approximates the native femoral stem-shaft angle of 135°. (*B*) AP radiograph of left hip resurfacing implant demonstrates measurement of the acetabular component inclination angle, typical values of which are 35° to 50°. (*C*) Cross-table lateral radiograph of left hip resurfacing implant demonstrates measurement of the acetabular anteversion angle, which typically measures between 5° and 20°.

metaphyseal stem is not commonly cemented or designed for fixation. It is present merely to guide the placement of the femoral implant during the surgical procedure. However, radiographically, the stem is an extremely useful tool in assessing implant stability. The stem has been likened to an "antennae" broadcasting the condition of the femoral head because of its extension. In examining the interface of the femoral stem and the bone of the native femoral neck, it is helpful to have a convention to describe the regions of interest. The most widely used convention is that used by Amstutz and colleagues.[13] In this methodology, the bone around the femoral stem is divided into 3 regions in the frontal plane: medial, lateral, and at the tip, the so-called peg zones. There may be a thin sclerotic line in all 3 peg zones that indicates a bony reaction to the metal stem, which does not indicate loosening. However, asymmetry along one of the peg zones is a sign of implant migration (**Fig. 3**).

The socket must also be carefully inspected for bone integration. Because all hip resurfacing acetabular components used today are designed for osseous integration, the presence of spot welds and bone trabeculae streaming to the implant interface are welcome signs. Radiolucencies around the socket may be thin and faint but are worrisome for failure to integrate (**Fig. 4**).

Impingement

Impingement, or abnormal contact of the bone on the arthroplasty, is another finding of conventional radiography. As opposed to total hip replacement, in which the neck is replaced by a prosthetic, hip resurfacing retains the native femoral neck, which can abut the acetabular component. In certain patients, this contact between the neck and rim of the socket can be seen as an indentation along the femoral neck; however, these patients typically are not symptomatic (**Fig. 5**).[14,15]

Neck narrowing

Neck narrowing, or neck thinning, is a phenomenon noted only in hip resurfacing. It is defined as a decrease in the femoral neck diameter measured at the implant-neck junction. In some studies, neck narrowing has been detected in 77% to 90% of resurfaced hips.[16,17] Neck narrowing is thought to be a benign process,

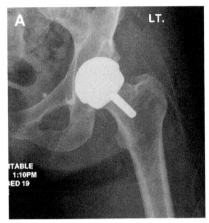
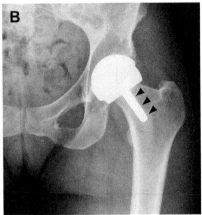

Fig. 3. (*A*) Immediate postoperative anteroposterior (AP) radiograph of left hip resurfacing implant. Notice the position of the stem within the native femoral bone. (*B*) AP radiograph of the same hip resurfacing after 2 years; notice the migration of the femoral stem into a lower stem-shaft angle (more varus). Furthermore, inspection of the peg zones reveals an asymmetric distance between the radiosclerotic line and the stem (*arrowheads*), indicating migration.

indicating remodeling because of alterations in bone loading (ie, stress shielding), and should be nonprogressive after 3 years (**Fig. 6**).

Heterotopic bone formation

Hip resurfacing may be more prone to forming heterotopic bone because of the larger surgical dissection necessary to perform the procedure. In some studies, significant heterotopic ossification was noted in up to 7% of patients undergoing the procedure.[13,18] The most common methodology

used in describing heterotopic ossification is the same as with total hip replacements, the classification by Brooker and colleagues.[19]

Stress fracture of the femoral neck

Femoral neck fracture is the most common reason for failure of hip resurfacing. Typically, it occurs within the first 3 months after operation and is evidenced by complete displacement at the implant-neck junction. Occasionally, if identified

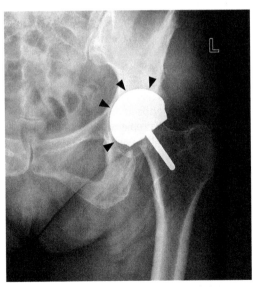

Fig. 4. Anteroposterior radiograph of left hip resurfacing demonstrates radiolucency around the circumference of the acetabular component (*arrowheads*). This socket was found to lack osseous integration at revision surgery.

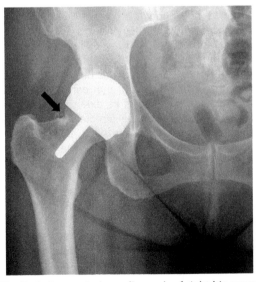

Fig. 5. Anteroposterior radiograph of right hip resurfacing demonstrates remodeling of the superolateral aspect of the femoral neck from impingement upon the prosthetic acetabular rim (*arrow*). Based on the location of this remodeling, impingement is likely to have occurred during abduction.

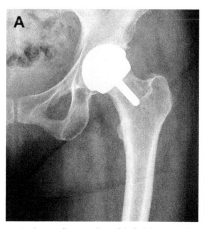
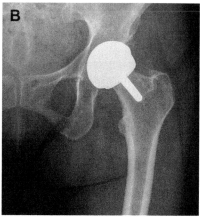

Fig. 6. Anteroposterior radiographs of left hip resurfacing immediately after surgery (*A*) and 3 years postoperatively (*B*). Note the decrease in diameter of the femoral neck at the implant-neck junction. This dimension did not further decrease after 1 year.

early, a fracture line can be detected, beginning from the tension side of the femoral neck at the head-neck junction. In this situation, immediate protected weight bearing may be able to prevent this type of fracture from displacement (**Fig. 7**).

ULTRASONOGRAPHY AND CT

Although conventional radiographs are useful for assessing the angle of inclination of the components, implant stability, and femoral neck narrowing, all of which may indicate potential implant failure,[20] radiographs may fail to detect or may grossly underestimate the presence of osteolysis.[7] Radiographs are also unable to detect soft tissue complications, including the presence of solid or cystic masses adjacent to the implant, which have been described as part of the spectrum of metal hypersensitivity.[1,3,5,21]

Adverse local tissue reaction (ALTR) is a relatively unique complication of MOM implants[22–24] and may manifest as solid or cystic groin lesions, which have been termed pseudotumors, as well as synovitis, bursitis, or periprosthetic osteolysis.[1,5,21] On biopsy or at revision surgery, the periprosthetic tissues are characterized by the presence of perivascular or diffuse infiltrates of B and T lymphocytes.[1,3,5] The incidence of such reactions after MOM hip resurfacing is unknown, but in larger retrospective studies, pseudotumors have been reported in up to 1% of patients at revision surgery[1,5] and are likely associated with high wear. The incidence may in fact be higher with certain designs and component malorientation. In addition, this reaction can occur in asymptomatic patients.[2,3,5]

Rarely, ALTR manifests as an allergic type of delayed hypersensitivity and is accompanied by the

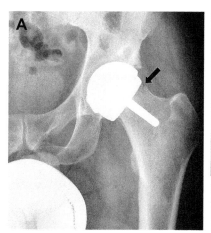
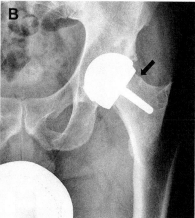

Fig. 7. Anteroposterior radiographs of left hip resurfacing at 6 weeks after operation (*A*). Note a femoral neck fracture at the superolateral implant-neck junction (*arrow, A*). With protection of weight bearing, subsequent radiographs at 1 year (*B*) demonstrated healing of the fracture (*arrow, B*).

histologic diagnosis of aseptic lymphocytic vasculitis associated lesions (ALVALs),[25] often with excessive necrosis but without significant wear-induced debris.

Ultrasonography is a useful screening tool to detect the presence of a soft tissue mass adjacent to an implant, which may indicate metal hypersensitivity.[1,5,6,26] Ultrasonography has also been used as a screening tool in asymptomatic patients to monitor for the presence of pseudotumors, which if present, may alert the clinician as to the need for closer monitoring for implant-related failure.[3] However, this technique is operator dependent and may not show deeper lesions optimally because of limited transmission.

CT can delineate solid or cystic masses in proximity to the implant[2,5,27] and has the additional benefit of providing bony detail to better delineate osseous complications such as osteolysis.[7] The use of CT with 3-dimensional (3D) measurement software has been suggested to allow better assessment of component alignment, which may be difficult to evaluate on axial CT or plain radiography because of obscuration of the acetabular component by the large diameter metal head.[2]

MRI

Given that most arthroplasties fail as a result of wear-induced synovitis, evaluation of the soft tissue envelope, and specifically the synovium, is warranted. Because of its multiplanar abilities, lack of ionizing radiation, and superior soft tissue contrast MRI is well suited in the evaluation of synovial reactions. However, the ferromagnetic nature of the cobalt-chromium components in conventional surface replacement generates a large degree of susceptibility artifacts. By definition, susceptibility artifact reflects the ability of the material to become magnetized when exposed to a high external magnetic field, such as that used in clinical MRI. The close juxtaposition of diamagnetic soft tissue with the relatively ferromagnetic arthroplasty components generates specific artifacts that affect the slice profile, yielding distortion in the slice direction, as well as frequency shifts and phase dispersion, which generate a "pile up" of signal with a characteristic high signal intensity focus at the metal–soft tissue interface (**Fig. 8**).

With appropriate pulse sequence modification, including strategies aimed to increase the strength of the magnetic gradients, reduction of this distortion in both the slice and the readout direction is achieved. The most effective clinically available means to modify the MRI protocols is the use of a wide receiver bandwidth. Although a high spatial resolution in the frequency direction does not necessarily diminish the artifact, it provides a better definition of the metal-induced distortion. Fast or turbo spin echo pulse sequences should be used to minimize signal loss secondary to diffusion. Caution should be used to avoid frequency-selective fat suppression or gradient echo techniques.

New pulse sequences are being developed to further minimize artifacts. Slice encoding for metal artifact correction is a modified pulse sequence that has been shown to reduce artifact generated by components.[28] More traditional view angle tilt pulse sequences have also been used, in which a slice-select gradient is reapplied during the readout, resulting in reregistration of in-plane and slice distortions.[29] Most recently, the multiple acquisition variable resonance image combination has been suggested, in which a 3D pulse sequence is acquired to reduce slice distortion,

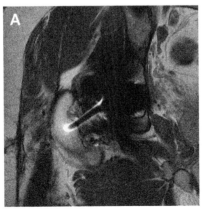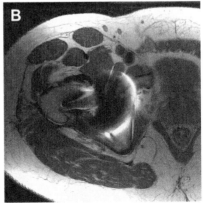

Fig. 8. Coronal (*A*) and axial (*B*) fast spin echo MRI of left hip resurfacing demonstrates the characteristic high signal intensity artifact at the metal–soft tissue interface. Note that the artifact is brighter than either fat or fluid because of the frequency shifts.

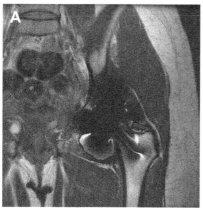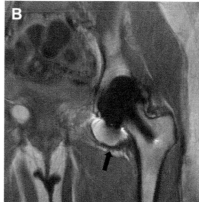

Fig. 9. Coronal fast spin echo (*A*) and coronal multiple acquisition variable resonance image combination proto-type sequence (*B*) MRI of left hip resurfacing. Note the significant reduction in artifact and improved visualization of the acetabulum, synovitis in the inferomedial recess (*arrow*), and periprosthetic soft tissues with the prototype sequence.

and multiple off-resonance images are obtained, compiled by a reconstruction algorithm that mark-edly reduces susceptibility shift (**Fig. 9**).[30,31] An optimized imaging protocol using commercially available nonprototype pulse sequences is sug-gested in **Table 1**.

Despite these challenges, effective artifact reduction has been generated. A previously re-ported cadaveric model of simulated osteolysis using conventional polyethylene on metal implants has demonstrated that MRI detects periacetabular osteolysis most accurately with a sensitivity of

Table 1
Sample protocol for MRI of hip arthroplasty

Timing Parameters	Axial FSE Body Coil	Coronal FMIR Body Coil	Coronal FSE Surface Coil	Axial FSE Surface Coil	Sagittal FSE Surface Coil
TR (ms)	4500–5500	4500	4500–5800	4500–5500	5500–6500
TE (ms)	21.4–32.0	18	24–30	24–30	23–30
TI (ms)	—	150	—	—	—
ETL	16–20	7–9	10–20	10–20	14–20
RBW (kHz)	83–100	83–100	83–100	83–100	83–100
FOV (cm)	32–36	34–36	18	17–19	18–20
Matrix	512 × 256	256 × 192	512 × 352	512 × (256 to 288)	512 × 352
Slice thickness (mm)	5	5	4	4	2.5–3
Interslice gap (mm)	0	0	0	0	0
NEX	4	2	4–5	4–5	4–5
Tailored RF	Yes	Yes	Yes	Yes	Yes
No phase wrap	Yes	Yes	Yes	Yes	Yes
Swap phase and frequency	Yes	Yes	Yes	Yes	Yes
Variable BW	Yes	Yes	Yes	Yes	Yes
Frequency direction	Anterior to posterior	Right to left	Right to left	Anterior to posterior	Anterior to posterior

Depending on the MRI system, the RBW may be reported as half-bandwidth (maximum frequency), so reported RBW of 62.5 is actually acquired at 125 Hz over the entire frequency range. For this table, to convert to Hz/pixel, use the following formula: (kHz × 2000)/512.

Abbreviations: BW, bandwidth; ETL, echo train length; FMIR, fast inversion recovery; FOV, field of view; FSE, fast spin echo; NEX, number of excitations; RBW, receiver bandwidth; RF, radiofrequency; TE, echo time; TI, inversion time; TR, repetition time.

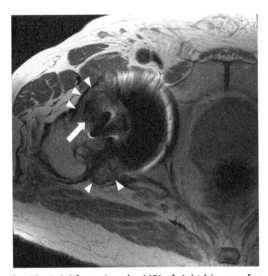

Fig. 10. Axial fast spin echo MRI of right hip resurfacing demonstrates expansion of the pseudocapsule with particulate debris (*arrowheads*) resulting in an indolent pattern of erosion of the anterior portion of the femoral neck (*arrow*).

95% compared with the sensitivities of 75% and 52% of optimized CT and standard oblique radiographs, respectively.[7] Further, MRI has been shown to better depict not only periacetabular bone loss but also the adverse synovial response, which may predate the presence of discernible bone loss on radiographs or MRI.[8]

To date, there are only limited data concerning the use of MRI in the assessment of MOM hip resurfacing implants. MRI has been shown to detect deep fluid collections or masses that are unable to be assessed with ultrasonography and has been used to clarify equivocal ultrasonographic

findings.[3,26] Reported findings on MRI have included large cystic or solid masses adjacent to the implant, which histologically have corresponded to ALVAL.[3,4] These findings often occur in the presence of normal-appearing radiographs, leading some investigators to recommend the early use of MRI in a patient presenting with pain after hip resurfacing.[4,5] The early application of MRI is useful because synovitis and/or osteolysis may be evaluated and tracked quantitatively using an optimized scanning protocol for longitudinal study.

Additional advantages of MRI include the ability to determine subtle erosion of the anterior portion of the femoral neck, possibly to be implicated in fatigue fractures adjacent to the thin femoral stem (**Fig. 10**). MRI can demonstrate dehiscence of the posterior capsule, which can allow for synovial expansion and preferential communication with the greater trochanteric bursa (**Fig. 11**). These large periprosthetic fluid collections, or the so-called pseudotumors, reflect wear-induced synovial disease that can decompress into the greater trochanteric, iliopsoas muscle, or subiliac bursae. Preferential expansion of the synovial envelope into associated bursae may result in neurovascular compression, either in the femoral or sciatic distributions, which can also be well demonstrated on MRI (**Fig. 12**).

MOM-induced synovial disease typically manifests as diffuse intermediate signal intensity debris. Areas of osteolysis are denoted as intermediate signal intensity replacement of bone marrow because of particulate matter replacing the normal high signal intensity of fatty marrow (**Fig. 13**). Eccentric wear of bone around the components can also result from capsular erosion by virtue of expansion of the synovial envelope,

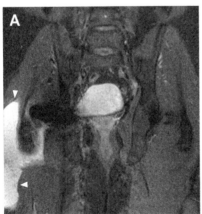
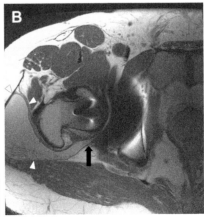

Fig. 11. Coronal inversion recovery (*A*) and axial fast spin echo (*B*) MRI of right hip resurfacing demonstrates extensive trochanteric bursitis (*arrowheads*) that communicates through the pseudocapsule at the posteromedial margin (*arrow, B*). Linear particulate debris within the collection indicates early wear-induced synovitis.

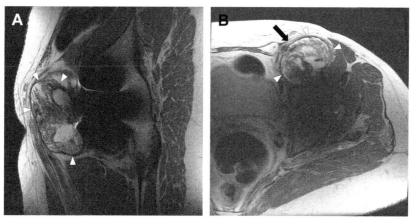

Fig. 12. Sagittal fast spin echo (FSE) (*A*) and axial FSE (*B*) MRI of left hip resurfacing in a patient who presented with an anterior hip mass. There is a complex fluid collection anterior to the prosthesis distending the iliopsoas bursa (*arrowheads*) and causing compression of the femoral neurovascular bundle (*arrow, B*).

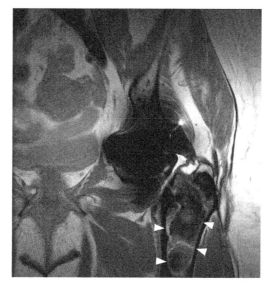

Fig. 13. Coronal fast spin echo MRI of left hip resurfacing demonstrates extensive femoral osteolysis with replacement of the normal marrow by intermediate signal intensity debris (*arrowheads*).

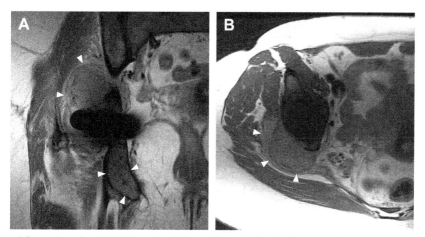

Fig. 14. Coronal fast spin echo (FSE) (*A*) and axial FSE (*B*) MRI of right hip resurfacing demonstrates large soft tissue mass posterolateral to the arthroplasty with destruction of the posterior margin of the acetabulum (*arrowheads*). The patient had a history of hemangiopericytoma; the findings represent metastatic disease.

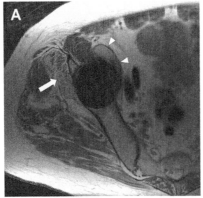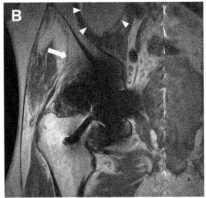

Fig. 15. Axial fast spin echo (FSE) (*A*) and coronal FSE (*B*) MRI of right hip resurfacing demonstrates subselective denervation effect in the gluteus minimus muscle resulting in moderate fatty infiltration (*arrow*). Also note large amount of fluid in the subiliac bursa (*arrowheads*).

causing pressure erosion with less particulate replacement of the normal marrow.

Atypical bone resorption should raise the concern of an alternative diagnosis, including tumoral replacement of bone, particularly in the setting of an appropriate patient history (**Fig. 14**). It is the authors' experience that osteolysis does not occur in the absence of any discernible synovitis or expansion of the pseudocapsule.[8]

In addition to the evaluation of bone loss and synovitis, MRI allows evaluation of the surrounding soft tissue envelope. The rotator cuff of the hip or hip abductors may be evaluated to identify insertional tendinosis and/or partial or complete tendon tears. Similar to the evaluation of the rotator cuff of the shoulder careful scrutiny of not only the integrity of the tendons but also the quality of the muscle should be undertaken, looking for subselective denervation effects, particularly in the gluteus minimus muscle, as well as severe atrophy in the setting of chronic tendon to bone failure (**Fig. 15**).

SUMMARY

Radiographic assessment remains the initial imaging mainstay for the evaluation of the painful surface replacement. In the setting of radiographs with equivocal or negative results, however, more advanced imaging is efficacious, including the use of optimized MRI. MRI allows for the quantitative and accurate assessment of intracapsular synovitis as well as the qualitative assessment of differential patterns of bone loss. In addition, MRI can detect eccentric or extensive synovial expansion that can result in neurovascular compression, accounting for sciatic or femoral nerve symptoms that may be erroneously attributed to spinal

pathologic condition. Furthermore, the surrounding soft tissue envelope may be evaluated, inclusive of the iliopsoas and hip abductor tendons.

REFERENCES

1. Campbell P, Shimmin A, Walter L, et al. Metal sensitivity as a cause of groin pain in metal-on-metal hip resurfacing. J Arthroplasty 2008;23(7):1080–5.
2. Hart AJ, Sabah S, Henckel J, et al. The painful metal-on-metal hip resurfacing. J Bone Joint Surg Br 2009;91(6):738–44.
3. Kwon YM, Ostlere SJ, McLardy-Smith P, et al. "Asymptomatic" pseudotumors after metal-on-metal hip resurfacing arthroplasty prevalence and metal ion study. J Arthroplasty 2010. [Epub ahead of print].
4. Ollivere B, Darrah C, Barker T, et al. Early clinical failure of the Birmingham metal-on-metal hip resurfacing is associated with metallosis and soft-tissue necrosis. J Bone Joint Surg Br 2009;91(8):1025–30.
5. Pandit H, Glyn-Jones S, McLardy-Smith P, et al. Pseudotumours associated with metal-on-metal hip resurfacings. J Bone Joint Surg Br 2008;90(7): 847–51.
6. Langton DJ, Jameson SS, Joyce TJ, et al. Early failure of metal-on-metal bearings in hip resurfacing and large-diameter total hip replacement: a consequence of excess wear. J Bone Joint Surg Br 2010;92(1):38–46.
7. Walde TA, Weiland DE, Leung SB, et al. Comparison of CT, MRI, and radiographs in assessing pelvic osteolysis: a cadaveric study. Clin Orthop Relat Res 2005;437:138–44.
8. Potter HG, Nestor BJ, Sofka CM, et al. Magnetic resonance imaging after total hip arthroplasty: evaluation of periprosthetic soft tissue. J Bone Joint Surg Am 2004;86(9):1947–54.

9. Johnson C. A new method for roentgenographic examination of the upper end of the femur. J Bone Joint Surg Am 1932;14:859–66.

10. Ghelman B, Kepler CK, Lyman S, et al. CT outperforms radiography for determination of acetabular cup version after THA. Clin Orthop Relat Res 2009; 467(9):2362–70.

11. Beaule PE, Lee JL, Le Duff MJ, et al. Orientation of the femoral component in surface arthroplasty of the hip. A biomechanical and clinical analysis. J Bone Joint Surg Am 2004;86(9):2015–21.

12. De Haan R, Pattyn C, Gill HS, et al. Correlation between inclination of the acetabular component and metal ion levels in metal-on-metal hip resurfacing replacement. J Bone Joint Surg Br 2008; 90(10):1291–7.

13. Amstutz HC, Beaule PE, Dorey FJ, et al. Metal-on-metal hybrid surface arthroplasty: two to six-year follow-up study. J Bone Joint Surg Am 2004;86(1): 28–39.

14. Ball ST, Schmalzried TP. Posterior femoroacetabular impingement (PFAI) - after hip resurfacing arthroplasty. Bull NYU Hosp Jt Dis 2009;67(2):173–6.

15. Gruen T, LeDuff M, Wisk L, et al. Long-term follow-up of the first 100 metal-on-metal hybrid hip resurfacing with repetitive impingement signs: radiographic assessment and clinical relevance. J Bone Joint Surg Am 2010;92(16):2663–71.

16. Hing CB, Young DA, Dalziel RE, et al. Narrowing of the neck in resurfacing arthroplasty of the hip: a radiological study. J Bone Joint Surg Br 2007; 89(8):1019–24.

17. Spencer S, Carter R, Murray H, et al. Femoral neck narrowing after metal-on-metal hip resurfacing. J Arthroplasty 2008;23(8):1105–9.

18. Rama KR, Vendittoli PA, Ganapathi M, et al. Heterotopic ossification after surface replacement arthroplasty and total hip arthroplasty: a randomized study. J Arthroplasty 2009;24(2):256–62.

19. Brooker AF, Bowerman JW, Robinson RA, et al. Ectopic ossification following total hip replacement. Incidence and a method of classification. J Bone Joint Surg Am 1973;55(8):1629–32.

20. Shimmin A, Beaule PE, Campbell P. Metal-on-metal hip resurfacing arthroplasty. J Bone Joint Surg Am 2008;90(3):637–54.

21. Nikolaou V, Bergeron SG, Huk OL, et al. Evaluation of persistent pain after hip resurfacing. Bull NYU Hosp Jt Dis 2009;67(2):168–72.

22. Christiansen K, Holmes K, Zilko PJ. Metal sensitivity causing loosened joint prostheses. Ann Rheum Dis 1980;39(5):476–80.

23. Hallab N, Merritt K, Jacobs JJ. Metal sensitivity in patients with orthopaedic implants. J Bone Joint Surg Am 2001;83(3):428–36.

24. Merritt K, Brown SA. Metal sensitivity reactions to orthopedic implants. Int J Dermatol 1981;20(2): 89–94.

25. Willert HG, Buchhorn GH, Fayyazi A, et al. Metal-on-metal bearings and hypersensitivity in patients with artificial hip joints. A clinical and histomorphological study. J Bone Joint Surg Am 2005;87(1): 28–36.

26. Toms AP, Nolan J, Barker T, et al. Early failure of a Birmingham resurfacing hip replacement with lymphoreticular spread of metal debris: pre-operative diagnosis with MR. Br J Radiol 2009;82(977): e87–91.

27. Boardman DR, Middleton FR, Kavanagh TG. A benign psoas mass following metal-on-metal resurfacing of the hip. J Bone Joint Surg Br 2006; 88(3):402–4.

28. Lu W, Pauly KB, Gold GE, et al. SEMAC: slice encoding for metal artifact correction in MRI. Magn Reson Med 2009;62(1):66–76.

29. Butts K, Pauly JM, Gold GE. Reduction of blurring in view angle tilting MRI. Magn Reson Med 2005;53(2): 418–24.

30. Koch KM, Lorbiecki JE, Hinks RS, et al. A multispectral three-dimensional acquisition technique for imaging near metal implants. Magn Reson Med 2009;61(2): 381–90.

31. Potter HG, Koff MF, Juluri V, et al. MR imaging of metal on metal surface replacements. New Orleans (LA): Hip Society/AAHKS Combined Specialty Day Meeting; 2010.

Complications After Metal-on-Metal Hip Resurfacing Arthroplasty

Harlan C. Amstutz, MD[a,*], Michel J. Le Duff, MA[a],
Patricia A. Campbell, PhD[b], Lauren E. Wisk, BS[c],
Karren M. Takamura, BA[a]

KEYWORDS

- Arthroplasty • Metal-on-metal • Hip resurfacing
- Complications

The new generation of hip metal-on-metal resurfacing arthroplasty (MMRA) devices have now been implanted for more than 13 years in the centers that initiated the return to this procedure.[1–6] Ten-year survivorship data for MMRA are currently being reported in international meetings, with the first publication of the results of 100 hips at 10 to 14 years showing an 88.5% survival rate (95% confidence interval, 80.2%–93.5%) and 100% in 28 hips with ideal bone (cysts <1 cm and component size >46).[7] These results represent a dramatic improvement over metal/polyethylene hip resurfacing introduced in the mid-1970s[8] and are comparable to total hip replacement (THR) survivorship in the Swedish registry for young patients implanted during the same period, before the introduction of alternate bearings.[9] During this period, an array of complications specific to hip resurfacing has been identified, and solutions to prevent these complications have been proposed with varying degrees of success. The cause of most complications is usually multifactorial and falls under the broad categories of patient selection, prosthetic design, and surgical technique.

This article determines the incidence and cause of the complications commonly associated with MMRA, as well as the proposed methods and their success in preventing those complications. A comprehensive review of the published literature related to MMRA of the hip was undertaken to this effect.

SEARCH STRATEGY AND CRITERIA

A systematic review of the available literature was performed to identify publications related to hip resurfacing arthroplasty. An electronic search of MEDLINE was conducted using the search engine of the US National Library of Medicine. We searched for articles published after January 1, 2000, in the English language. Alternate keywords such as surface arthroplasty and surface replacement were added to the search because the term resurfacing, now predominantly accepted to describe the procedure, was not used systematically

One or more of the authors (H.C.A.) has consultancies and patent/licensing arrangements with Wright Medical Technologies Inc.

The institution of the authors (H.C.A., M.J.L.) has received funding from Wright Medical Technologies, Inc and the St Vincent Medical Center Foundation.

Work performed at the Joint Replacement Institute at Saint Vincent Medical Center, Los Angeles, CA.

[a] Joint Replacement Institute at Saint Vincent Medical Center, The S. Mark Taper Building, 2200 West Third Street, Suite 400, Los Angeles, CA 90057, USA

[b] J. Vernon Luck Research Center at Orthopaedic Hospital, 2400 South Flower Street, Los Angeles, CA 90057, USA

[c] Department of Population Health Sciences, School of Medicine and Public Health, University of Wisconsin, 610 North Walnut Street, WARF Office 558, Madison, WI 53726, USA

* Corresponding author.

E-mail address: harlanamstutz@dochs.org

orthopedic.theclinics.com

until after a sizable part of the related literature had already been published. We excluded expert opinions and editorial publications. We retained the studies that provided information about the incidence, etiology, or prevention of the type of complication reviewed in each subsection. Finally, we searched for relevant work in the bibliographies provided in recent review articles to identify additional studies that did not appear in the systematic search.

FEMORAL NECK FRACTURE
Incidence of Femoral Neck Fractures

To assess the worldwide incidence of femoral neck fracture after modern hip resurfacing, we collected data from the reports providing this information since 2005 and selected the most recent when several reports were published based on the same series of patients.[1,5,10–29] Our computations yielded a 1.69% incidence of femoral neck fracture (range, 0%–9.2%) for a global cohort of 10,381 cases, including 3497 from the Australian Hip Registry (**Table 1**).[25]

Etiology of Femoral Neck Fractures

The variability reflects the influence of surgeon experience, criteria for patient selection, component design, and surgical technique. Campbell and colleagues[30] have performed extensive studies of failed MMSA. Failures ranged from 1 week to several years postoperatively. Of the 98 failures submitted for analysis, the most common cause of failure was femoral neck fracture (32%). Most of these fractures occurred within 2 months of surgery, but in 7 cases, the average time to fracture was 15 months. The procedure of resurfacing itself is thought to increase strains in the lateral aspect of the femoral neck and the lesser trochanter region.[31–33] Shimmin and Back[25] reviewed the resurfacing experience within the Australian National Registry of joint replacements, which includes predominately Birmingham hip resurfacing (BHR) (Smith and Nephew, Inc, Memphis, TN, USA) types, and reported that fractures of the femoral neck were twice as likely in women than men and were more prevalent when the femoral implant was placed in the varus. The effect of femoral component positioning on the potential risk of neck fracture was further studied by the finite element analysis or cadaver studies, and the consensus is that valgus placement is recommended to avoid femoral neck fracture,[34–37] although Vail and colleagues[38] suggest that small deviations from the anatomic placement of the component result in high localized stresses on the femoral neck.

The multifactorial nature of this complication was first highlighted by Amstutz and colleagues,[39] who showed that most fractures that occurred in hips had more than 1 possible cause. Fractures that occurred early, within 2 months, were located at the neck component junction (subcapital), and the fracture of the hip, which occurred later (at 20 months post operatively), was located within the femoral head (intracapital) at the junction of viable and nonviable or repairing bone.

Notching has been reported in both fractured and successful resurfacings.[27] Occasionally, stress fractures occurring under MMRA components have been reported to heal if noted early and if the hip is protected by a period of non–weight-bearing.[40] Bone undergoing repair following stress fracture is a site of weakness for eventual fatigue failure.

Several incomplete (premonitory) and complete subcapital fractures were found unexpectedly by Campbell and colleagues[41] after retrieval in resurfacing revised for pain or femoral migration (**Fig. 1**). This case also illustrates the danger of over-pressurization of cement into the dome, which has been observed more often in those devices in which there is minimal or no cement mantle. Many of these failures can be considered to have a dual-phase failure mode; the original trauma to the bone occurs at surgery, but the actual failure process takes place several weeks or months later. Histologic analysis of the short-term fractures showed that the break occurred through areas of healing cancellous and cortical bone at the component/neck region. Similar findings were reported by Morlock and colleagues[42] after the analysis of fracture patterns and histologic findings among 141 femoral resurfacing failures. Early fractures were associated with uncovered reamed bone and microfractures, with associated healing. The investigators speculated that failure occurred when forces and moments on the bone exceeded the strength of the weakened bone. Pseudoarthrotic features were commonly found within the components and were attributed to a 2-time fracture time line. The cause of the initial injury was suggested to be either trauma or surgically induced damage, such as excessively high implantation forces necessary to seat tight femoral prosthetic devices, leaving little or no room to express excess cement.[43,44] In addition, the heat generated by the curing cement is related to the quantity of cement present under the femoral component, and an excessive amount may lead to thermal necrosis.[30,45] However, the use of lesser trochanteric suction, copious pulsatile lavage, and an early reduction of the hip reduces the temperature increase to physiologic levels at

Table 1
Recent publications (2005 or later) reporting femoral neck fracture rates

Authors	Journal	Year	Implant	Surgeons	Number of Hips	Number of Neck Fractures	Percentage
Madhu et al[17]	J Arthroplasty	2010	BHR	1 surgeon	117	5	4.3
Jameson et al[14]	J Bone Joint Surg Br	2010	ASR	1 surgeon	214	4	1.9
Ollivere et al[23]	Int Orthop	2009	BHR	1 surgeon	104	0	0
Khan et al[15]	J Arthroplasty	2009	BHR	Multicenter	679	11	1.6
Beaulé et al[10]	J Arthroplasty	2009	Conserve® Plus	1 surgeon	116	0	0
O'Neill et al[22]	Bull of NYU Hosp Jt Dis	2009	5 designs	Multicenter	250	4	1.6
Steffen et al[27]	J Arthroplasty	2009	4 designs	5 surgeons	842	15	1.8
Amstutz and Le Duff[1]	J Arthroplasty	2008	Conserve® Plus	1 surgeon	1000	10	1.0
Della Valle et al[12]	Clin Orthop Relat Res	2008	BHR	Multicenter	537	10	1.9
Heilpern et al[13]	J Bone Joint Surg Br	2008	BHR	1 surgeon	110	1	0.9
Kim et al[16]	J of Arthroplasty	2008	Conserve® Plus	Multicenter	200	2	1.0
Witzleb et al[29]	Eur J Med Res	2008	BHR	1 surgeon	300	1	0.3
McAndrew et al[18]	Hip Int	2007	BHR	Multicenter	180	8	2.2
Mont et al[19]	Clin Orthop Relat Res	2007	Conserve® Plus	Multicenter	1016	27	2.7
Marker et al[20]	J Arthroplasty	2007	Conserve® Plus	1 surgeon	550	14	2.5
Nishii et al[21]	J Arthroplasty	2007	BHR	1 surgeon	50	1	2.0
Siebel et al[26]	JEIM	2006	ASR	1 surgeon	300	5	1.7
Vail et al[28]	Clin Orthop Relat Res	2006	Conserve® Plus	1 surgeon	57	1	1.8
Pollard et al[24]	J Bone Joint Surg Br	2006	BHR	1 surgeon	63	3	4.8
Shimmin & Back[25]	J Bone Joint Surg Br	2005	BHR	Multicenter	3497	50	1.4
Treacy et al[5]	J Bone Joint Surg Br	2005	BHR	1 surgeon	144	1	0.7
Cutts et al[11]	Hip Int	2005	Cormet	5 surgeons	65	6	9.2
Total	—			—	10,381	175	1.69

Abbreviation: BHR, Birmingham hip resurfacing.

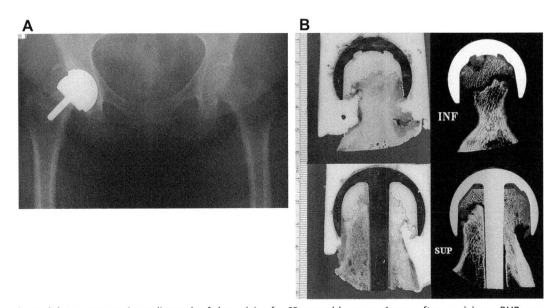

Fig. 1. (*A*) Anteroposterior radiograph of the pelvis of a 63-year-old woman 1 year after receiving a BHR resurfacing device. The acetabular component is loose, and that was the reason for scheduling the revision. (*B*) Cut sections and microradiographs of the femoral head. Cement was occupying 52% and 48% (overpressurized) of the posterior (*top*) and middle sections (*bottom*), respectively. The femoral head demonstrated a previously unrecognized incomplete fracture at the junction of the deeply penetrated cement, but the head was mostly viable and vascular.

the bone-cement interface[46] as does the use of a manual bone-cement application.[47,48] However, these studies have not been confirmed histologically.

The Role of Vascularity

Little and colleagues[49] proposed that fractures occurred because the femoral head bone was devascularized and weakened during the surgery, specifically because resurfacing was performed through the posterior approach, which is thought to destroy the extraosseous blood supply to the femoral head. This proposition was based on the histologic observation of extensive background necrosis among 12 of 13 failed resurfacings from a cohort of 377, mostly BHR, implants from the investigators' institution. However, there are no other retrieval studies that have shown such a high proportion of necrosis, and histologic sections showing the degree of necrosis have not been published. Further, these determinations were made on a single section, which may not be representative of the entire femoral head. Blood flow in the femoral head has been studied by the same Oxford group using oxygen/nitrogen saturations[50] and by others using laser Doppler flowmetry technique.[51–53] These studies showed that dislocation and subsequent tissue dissection during the posterior approach led to a marked

reduction in blood supply to the sampled areas of the femoral head. Because the volume of the bone sampled by the probe was not disclosed, it is not clear if the measurements reflect a similar loss of blood supply throughout the femoral head because of the limited areas of sampling. Khan and colleagues,[54] using cefuroxime, a cephalosporin routinely given for antibiotic prophylaxis during hip surgery, as an indicator of the blood supply to the femoral head, reported that the posterolateral approach was associated with a significant reduction in the blood supply compared with the transgluteal approach. These studies are inconclusive in our view because the degree of avascularity has not yet been correlated with the incidence of femoral neck fractures. Recent studies on resurfaced femoral heads with positron emission tomographic (PET) scans reported good bone viability,[55] but it is not clear if this is due to preservation of the original supply or reestablishment of temporarily compromised vascularity. Because the incidence of femoral neck fracture is very low and varies among surgeons, the significance of these studies remains controversial. In a PET scan study limited by a less number of subjects, Ullmark and colleagues[56] found 3 cases of head necrosis at 1 year of follow-up and concluded that the delayed onset of the necrosis did not support the hypothesis of surgically damaged bone caused by avascularity. In addition, Hananouchi and colleagues[57] showed that the intraosseous vascular network around the head-neck junction is not compromised sufficiently after resurfacing to induce complete avascularity. Because the incidence of femoral neck fracture is very low and varies among surgeons, the significance of these studies remains controversial. The amount of extreme internal rotation and duration of that position during acetabular preparation and biologic variability among patients are also possible contributing factors.

Although diminution of blood flow would be anticipated in normal, nonarthritic femoral heads after the section of the lateral circumflex artery, we have invariably observed intraoperative gross vascularity with bleeding surfaces from the arthritic head. Because some attenuation would be anticipated even in the arthritic hip, this bleeding suggests that a hypervascular state occurs within the osteoarthritic hip. This observed hyperemia has been verified with PET scan studies by Forrest and colleagues.[55] Blood supply to the osteoarthritic femoral head must occur by anastomosis and collateral circulation through the neck to the femoral head because the osteophytes often associated with the osteoarthritic disease generally occlude the branches from the medial circumflex artery, which normally enter the head at the head-neck junction.

Extensive histologic analyses of failed resurfaced femoral heads by Campbell and colleagues[30] have demonstrated some areas of dead bone in short-term retrievals with surrounding new bone formation, but rarely whole head necrosis. These healing areas of necrotic bone generally have ample reserve to sustain overall viability.

There is a concern that the prevalence of femoral neck fractures in women may increase with advancing age as compared with that in men. Hip resurfacing has been shown to preserve the bone mineral density (BMD) of the proximal femur over time after surgery, when the operated hip is compared with the contralateral hip.[58] Also, BMD is better preserved after resurfacing than after a conventional total hip arthroplasty (THA).[59] Age itself is not a predictor of femoral neck fracture after hip resurfacing.[60,61] No evidence exists in the literature that women who underwent resurfacing sustain a nontraumatic neck fracture in their lifetime. According to the North American Menopause Society, postmenopausal women who are older than 65 years or weigh less than 57.73 kg (127 lb) are most at risk for osteoporosis.[62] Ahlborg and colleagues[63] showed that postmenopausal women experience an increase in skeletal size as a result of periosteal apposition, which at least partially compensates for the potential decrease in bone strength from the loss of bone density.

Based on the literature,[63–67] certain physiologic changes that occur naturally with aging can in fact provide positive bone modifications that may reduce the risk of fracture and benefit the outcome of the prosthesis. Further follow-up is necessary to determine whether our belief that well-performed hip resurfacings in women with osteoarthritis are not vulnerable to subsequent fracture with advancing age.

In summary, it seems that most causes of femoral fractures are multifactorial and usually related to deficiencies in technique, whereas the significance of vascular changes remains controversial.

Prevention of Femoral Neck Fractures

Most surgeons continue to use the posterior approach because it is more direct, and optimal component orientation is facilitated.[68] The advantages of other approaches introduced mostly to preserve the blood supply have not been conclusively demonstrated. Notches should be avoided, and the component needs to be fully seated. Performing cylindrical reaming in stages with a system allowing the pin to be moved up until the last ream will prevent any risk of notching.[69] The preservation of the anterior osteophyte, when present, has been suggested because this osteophyte may play a supporting role in the overall strength of the neck. This preservation can be achieved by orienting the femoral component more anteriorly on the neck and inserting it slightly posterior to anterior.[68,70] Several surgeons have proposed other approaches to minimize the potential risk of loss of blood supply: the Ganz approach with a trochanteric flip[10] or an anterior approach.[71–73] Although the exposure is excellent with the trochanteric flip, there has been a high incidence of trochanteric nonunion (10%) often associated with local bursitis, requiring removal of the screws.[10] The exposure obtained with the anterior approach, we believe, is more limited and may not be suitable for all patients. However, it is generally recommended that surgeons learning the resurfacing technique should use the approach with which they are most familiar.

Femoral component alignment may be a factor in the prevention of femoral neck fractures, and the use of navigation has been recommended as a surgical tool to optimize orientation.[74,75]

Several investigators recommend avoiding high-load physical activities during the time needed for the bone to remodel around the prosthesis,[76,77] but this recommendation also warrants further investigation.

ASEPTIC LOOSENING
Incidence of Femoral Component Loosening

The incidence of femoral loosening in most reported series with a 5-year follow-up is low, ranging from 0% to 1.3%.[5,15,21,78,79] However, these series were essentially composed of patients with predominately large component sizes and small cystic defects. A 2% rate of femoral loosening was reported in a series of all comers with a mean follow-up of 5.6 years.[1]

A higher incidence of femoral component loosening (5 of 104) has been reported at a mean follow-up of 4.3 years in a series of hips with osteonecrosis.[80] In this report and 2 other series, the surgeons accepted no more than 30% of necrotic involvement in the femoral head; Revell and colleagues[81] reported 97.3% femoral component survival at 6.1 years, and Mont and colleagues[82] mentioned 1 femoral loosening in 42 hips at a mean follow-up of 41 months. In contrast, despite an absence of restrictions on the degree of necrotic involvement acceptable in the femoral head, a femoral survivorship of 97% at 10 years was recently reported, with only 2 cases of femoral loosening in 85 hips and none in surgeries performed after 1997.[83] These rather remarkable results are believed to be the result of a thorough removal of all the yellow necrotic

bone with a high-speed burr in hips with osteonecrosis, combined with bone cleansing, drying, and optimized cementing technique. As the results of longer follow-ups become available on the series of patients with hip osteonecrosis, it becomes apparent that the indications for metal-on-metal resurfacing are expanding because it provides a much more reliable pain relief than hemiresurfacing.[83,84] To obviate femoral loosening, Gross and Back[85] reported promising midterm results in a small group of patients with an uncemented femoral resurfacing component, although their cohort still experienced only a 78.9% survival rate at 7 years because of other causes, including 2 cases of acetabular loosening. Also, Lilikakis and colleagues[86] showed early success with the same cementless design in a series of 66 patients (70 hips).

Etiology of Femoral Component Loosening

The main risk factors for femoral loosening are small component size and femoral head defects larger than 1 cm (**Fig. 2**), identified in a 2004 publication of the results for 400 resurfaced hips,[87] and a low body mass index (BMI).[88] Aseptic loosening of the femoral component is a time-dependant process, for which an early detection can be helpful. Several methods have been proposed, including measurement of plain radiographs,[89] Einzel-Bild-Röntgen-analyze (EBRA),[90] and radiostereophotogrammetry (RSA).[91] However, none of these methods provide the means to reliably

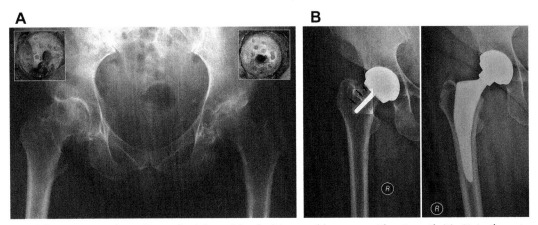

Fig. 2. (*A*) Anteroposterior radiograph of the pelvis of a 51-year-old woman with osteoarthritis. Note the extensive femoral head defects left after removal of the cystic material. Not all of the cystic material was removed from the head, and there was less-than-optimal cleaning and drying, leading to less-than-optimal initial fixation. The stem was also not cemented in, as would be our practice today with cysts of this size and small component size. (*B*) One hundred and eleven months after resurfacing. The 38-mm femoral component is loose, as shown by the large radiolucency that was first observed around the metaphyseal stem at 12 months. The well-fixed acetabular component (abduction 43° and anteversion 12.6°) was retained at revision surgery and matched with a unipolar head of appropriate diameter. (Her serial ion studies were consistently normal for a bilateral resurfacing, with cobalt, 3.4 ppb, and chromium, 7.1 ppb, at 76 months postoperation.)

study component migration on a large series. RSA is not practical to use in a routine clinical setting, and EBRA or plain radiographic measurement is reliable only if the radiographs compared present the same femoral rotation (which is rarely the case in any series of radiographs), because they are 2-dimensional solutions measuring a 3-dimensional phenomenon.

Other investigators have suggested that the inner geometry of the femoral component was associated with potential debonding and stress shielding or stress concentration, which might adversely affect survivorship.[77,92–95] Although legitimate in theory, these claims remain to be confirmed by the rapid fall of survivorship in a large series of MMRA, and no such report has been published so far.

A fibrous interface is to be avoided because movement between the bone and the cement cannot be tolerated.[96] Retrieval analyses of long-term resurfacings show variable amounts of bone remodeling. Areas of bone thinning are often accompanied by solidification of the bone elsewhere, which can provide remarkable durability despite major bone loss.[30] This process highlights the remarkable adaptive capability of the human femoral head to withstand the damage induced by resurfacing.

Prevention of Femoral Component Loosening

Amstutz and colleagues[97] showed the effectiveness of modified surgical techniques on the rate of femoral component loosening, especially in patients with risk factors. A review of the intraoperative photos of the prepared femoral head in conjunction with a component retrieval analysis led to substantial improvements in component fixation techniques (**Fig. 3**).

The evolution of the surgical technique and its effects on prosthetic survival have previously been published[1,68,70,97] and follow 4 principles:

1. Thorough cleaning of the femoral head. This includes the removal of any cystic material with a high-speed burr and cleansing with lavage.
2. Maximization of the area for fixation. This includes the use of multiple small drill holes performed with a one-eighth-of-an-inch drill bit, rather than fewer larger holes.
3. Drying of the femoral head before cementation. This includes the use of suction to keep the bone dry until the acrylic has set and is also facilitated by the use of CO_2 applied with the Carbojet (Kinamed Inc, Camarillo, CA, USA) as shown in **Fig. 3**A.
4. Cementation with a uniform cement mantle of about 1 mm and a penetration of 1 to 3 mm.[41] A uniform pressurization is achievable with regular acrylic in a doughy stage rather than top-down pressurization of low-viscosity cement, which leads to overpressurization of the dome. Timing is critical, and the 1-mm gap allows extrusion of excess cement without overpenetrating the proximal bone (see **Fig. 1**).[47,98]

In addition, the effectiveness of cementing the metaphyseal stem for small component sizes and hips with large defects was recently demonstrated.[99] The cementation of the femoral stem adds surface area for fixation, although it

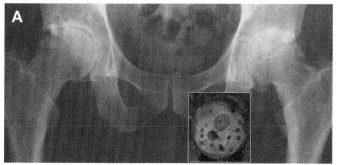 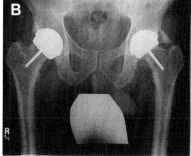

Fig. 3. (*A*) Anteroposterior radiograph of the pelvis of a 54-year-old man with bilateral osteoarthritis. The inset shows the femoral head after preparation (second generation). Note the complete removal of all cystic material, how clean and dry the bone is, and the abundance of drill holes in the chamber and dome portions of the head, particularly in sclerotic bone. (*B*) Seven years after left staged hip resurfacing and 5 years after right staged hip resurfacing, the patient's University of California at Los Angeles hip scores are 8 (*left*) and 10 (*right*) for pain, 10 for walking, 10 for function, and 7 for activity. Note the absence of heterotopic bone formation on the right hip, which was treated with our radiotherapy protocol in contrast to the left hip for which only indomethacin was used.

could potentially increase stress shielding within the femoral head.[100] However, clinical results of hips implanted with this technique currently show an absence of femoral component loosening.[99] In this study, caution about the practice of impact sports was raised for patients with a cemented metaphyseal stem because cement has a different modulus of elasticity than the bone, and repetitive impact may initiate micromotion between bone and cement and contribute to a loosening process.

Incidence of Acetabular Component Loosening

All currently available hip resurfacing systems use a cementless acetabular component. The superiority of cementless acetabular fixation for MMRA was clearly demonstrated by Beaulé and colleagues.[101] The reported incidence of acetabular component loosening is low for most cementless designs. At a mean follow-up of 5 years, Hing and colleagues[78] reported 1 (0.4%) aseptic acetabular component loosening from a series of 230 BHR resurfacings. O'Neill and colleagues[22] reported 2 (0.8%) cases of acetabular component loosening in a series of 250 hips resurfaced by 5 surgeons using a variety of modern-generation resurfacing devices, and Amstutz and Le Duff[1] reported no acetabular component loosening in 1000 hips at a mean follow-up of 5.6 years (range, 1–11 years). This issue contains the first report of radiographic studies specifically addressing the performance of 1-piece metal-on-metal acetabular components used in hip resurfacing, with a 5-year minimum follow-up (see the article by Ball and colleagues elsewhere in this issue for further exploration of this topic). Using radiographic evidence of loss of acetabular fixation (complete radiolucency covering all 3 zones), this study reported a Kaplan-Meier survival estimate of the acetabular component of 99.6% at 5 years and 97.6% at 10 years. Kim and colleagues[16] reported 10 (5%) cases of acetabular loosening in a multicenter series of 200 hips and attributed this result to the surgeons' learning curve.

In contrast, several reports raise concern relating a high incidence of acetabular loosening with 2 designs. Cutts and colleagues[11] used the Cormet device (Corin Medical Ltd, Cirencester, UK) and reported 4 cases of acetabular component loosening in 65 hips (6.2%). This report was corroborated by Dixon and colleagues,[102] who reported a 10% aseptic loosening rate at 5 years with the same design. Long and colleagues[103] reported a high short-term failure rate (mean, 1.6 years) in 29 of 207(14%) hips implanted with Durom monoblock cups (Zimmer, Warsaw, IN, USA) used with conventional stem-type THA, although a group of surgeons from Montreal had better results in the use of this acetabular component for resurfacing.[104,105] This device has now been withdrawn from the US market by the manufacturer. At the very least, it seems that the surgical technique for this system was critical and required that the acetabular preparation be sufficiently deep to completely seat the component within the acetabular walls.

Historically, a higher rate of acetabular component loosening has been reported in patients with developmental dysplasia of the hip (DDH) treated with hip resurfacing.[106] Several reports show that the current acetabular component designs perform well in this challenging etiologic group,[21,107,108] whether adjunct fixation is used[109] or not.[110,111] However, 1 center found a greater rate of acetabular component loosening in patients with DDH compared with patients with primary osteoarthritis.[112]

Prevention of Acetabular Component Loosening

Surgical technique is key to both the initial and enduring fixation of the acetabular component. The facility to achieve initial fixation varies with the different designs that have a variable amount of hemispherical coverage (165°–180°), roughness of coatings (porous beads of various sizes, plasma spray), and different methods of preparation and insertion (instruments and techniques) as shown in **Table 2**.

Results vary with the design used and the experience and expertise of the surgeon. Because of these variations and the lack of published radiographic data on all but 1 design, it is not possible to determine the true significance and effects of all the different features between designs on the ability to obtain initial and enduring fixation.

The surgical technique recommended for the implantation of the Conserve® Plus socket (Wright Medical Technology, Inc, Arlington, TN, USA) has been described in the peer-reviewed literature[68] and has some universal applicability. The careful assessment of the sphericity and interference fit of the created acetabular cavity are extremely important in achieving initial stability with a monoblock socket where there is no adjunctive fixation system. In addition, the rim must be free of soft tissue, which may be dragged into the component bone interface and decrease the contact area for ingrowth, depending on the system used. After insertion, it is essential to check the rigidity of the fixation by rocking the pelvis with the bayonet inserted in the locked position.

Table 2
Technical characteristics of the acetabular components for the currently used hip resurfacing designs

System	Date	Process	Heat Treatment	Clearance (μ)	Coverage (°)	Shape	Surface	Shell Thickness (mm)	Instrumentation
		Bearing			**Acetabular Component**				
Conserve® Plus	1996	Wrought or cast (Fem) Cast (Acet)	HIP, SA	100–220	170 outside, 170 inside, constant for all sizes	Truncated hemisphere	Sintered Co-Cr beads (0.3-mm diameter; 0.75-mm thickness) ± HA	3.5 or 5.5	Rigid bayonet coupling; inserter removable; capacity to reattach, extract, and reimplant component
BHR	1997	Cast	None	260 (size 54)	180 outside, 164 inside, decreasing with smaller sizes	Truncated hemisphere	Co-Cr beads (0.9–1.3 mm) cast-in + HA	3 rim, 6 dome	Instrument for insertion attached by wires, and once cut, extraction no longer possible
Cormet 2000	1997	Cast	HIP, SA	150–400[a]	—	Equatorial expansion	Ti-VPS + HA	3 and 4 (2 cups per head)	Inserter fits into cup face recesses, no extractor
Durom	2001	Wrought/forged	None	150 range unknown	165 inside, constant for all sizes	Truncated hemisphere	Ti-VPS	4	Inserter fits into cup face recesses, no extractor
ASR	2003	Cast	HIP, SA	100 midrange size[b]	170 outside, 156 inside, decreasing with smaller sizes	Truncated hemisphere	Sintered Co-Cr beads + HA	3–5	Inserter fits in recesses inside the socket, reducing head coverage
ReCap (Biomet)	2004	Cast	None	240 for size 46[c]	180 outside, inside unknown	Hemisphere	Ti-VPS ± HA	4	Equatorial diameter 2 mm greater than dome; inserter fits into cup face recesses, no extractor

Abbreviations: Acet, acetabular component; Fem, femoral component; HA, hydroxyapatite coated; HIP, hot isostatic pressing; SA, solution annealed; Ti-VPS, Titanium-Vacuum Plasma Spray.

[a] From the Corin Executive Summary of the IDE study results, FDA Web site. Available at: http://www.accessdata.fda.gov/cdrh_docs/pdf5/P050016b.pdf.

[b] Isaac G, Thompson J, Williams S, et al. Proc IMech, vol 220, Part H. J Engineering in Medicine 2006.

[c] Kretzer JP, Heisel C. Comparison of the macro- and microstructure of resurfacing hip implants. In: Sixth Combined Meeting of the Orthopaedic Research Society. Honolulu, October 20–24, 2007.

ADVERSE LOCAL TISSUE REACTIONS TO WEAR PRODUCTS

There is considerable concern regarding the potential biologic reactivity to metal particles and the presently unknown long-term effects of exposure to cobalt and chromium ions released from metal-on-metal articulating surfaces. The term adverse local tissue reaction (ALTR) was first proposed by Schmalzried[113] to include all adverse responses proceeding from both mechanical and biologic sources. The study of ALTR relies heavily on the analysis of the presence of metal ions produced by the bearing surfaces in the patient's blood or urine. There is still much to determine regarding the optimal methodology to conduct these studies. Whole blood analysis has its proponents,[114] whereas serum-based studies find their justification in a publication by Walter and colleagues.[115] Exercise-related elevation of plasma cobalt levels may be used as a tool to monitor bearing performance more precisely than baseline measurements.[116,117]

Incidence of ALTR

Most publications on this topic tend to describe the observed phenomena, but few actually provide information on their incidence. Pandit and colleagues[118] estimated that about 1% of the patients treated with MMRA develop a pseudotumor within 5 years. In later publications, the same group of researchers reported a 4% rate of revision at 8 years because of the development of pseudotumors[119] and pointed out the difficulty of successfully revising these cases.[120,121] They have also identified gender and age as having significant independent influences on revision rates for pseudotumors and cautioned against using metal-on-metal resurfacings in women younger than 40 years.[119] Subsequently, this group reported the incidence of asymptomatic pseudotumors to be 4.4% in a study of 158 patients with metal-on-metal hip resurfacings.[122] Their study found significantly higher cobalt and chromium concentrations in both serum and hip aspirate fluid in patients who developed the pseudotumors. In contrast, Malviya and Holland[123] reported a lower rate of revision at 0.15% due to pseudotumors in a series of 670 hips with up to 10 years of follow-up. Jameson and colleagues[14] and Langton and colleagues[124] recently reported a 2.8% and a 3.4% rate, respectively, of wear-related failures with the ASR cup (Depuy Orthopaedics, Warsaw, IN, USA) and mentioned their decision to no longer implant this device in small sizes. This device has subsequently been recalled worldwide.

Etiology of ALTR

In recent publications, ALTRs include adverse periprosthetic tissue reactions,[118,119,123,125] metal allergy,[126,127] and metallosis.[128] With the large diversity of reactions reported in the literature, a classification scheme would be helpful to apprehend the complexity of the observed phenomena and is proposed here to include all of the reported types of reactions:

ALTR I: Osteolysis caused by wear but without soft tissue local fluid or solid mass
ALTR II: Local fluid or solid mass secondary to high wear
ALTR III: Allergy or hypersensitivity without high wear.

These reactions can be variously related to the materials used. Devices using a low carbon content produce greater wear than bearings made with a high carbon content, whereas the manufacturing process (cast vs wrought) seems to have little effect on the wear of high-carbon components.[129] Diametral clearance has been shown to greatly affect component wear in vitro, particularly with large-size bearings.[130,131] The diameter of the bearing itself is also an important factor, and larger component sizes have been shown to produce less wear during the bedding-in phase[130,132] because a "continuous fluid film" lubrication mode is more readily achieved with large bearings.[131,133] More investigation led to the identification of the mixed nature (nano-crystalline and organic) of the contacting surfaces in sliding metal-on-metal bearings.[134] However, Clarke and colleagues[135] found higher metal ion levels in a group of patients who underwent MMRA compared with a group of patients who received 28-mm metal-on-metal THA devices, whereas other studies with a similar design found no difference between the 2 groups.[136–138] The wear-in (or bedding-in) phase of the bearings that happens during the first million cycles was confirmed in longitudinal studies of metal ion levels in patients implanted with resurfacing devices.[139–141] However, Heisel and colleagues[141] found that in vivo ion data show a slow increase, which is different from wear simulator data and probably related to the body's regulating functions. However, these measurements were made in a series of patients with ASR components, in which prosthetic size and component orientation were not included. This series was the earliest report of higher wear with this device.

The replacement of a femoral head to articulate with a previously used cup generates a new wear-in phase but of a lesser magnitude than the original bedding-in.[142,143] The particles generated by metal-on-metal bearings (in vivo and in hip simulators) are an order of magnitude smaller than polyethylene particles,[144] but still provide a large surface area for corrosion.[145] Thus, in addition to metal particulates, corrosion products are likely to induce local tissue reactions.[127,146] Davies and colleagues[147] pointed out the difference in the patterns and types of inflammation caused in the periprosthetic tissues of metal-on-metal and metal-polyethylene devices. Component orientation with metal-on-metal just as with alumina-alumina bearings is more critical than with metal-polyethylene bearings, and low coverage angles may be the result of excessive lateral opening, anteversion, or a combination of both and related to higher wear rates.

Several methods of detection are being used to assess the causes and consequences of high wear. They include computed tomography and EBRA[148] to assess component orientation, metal ion measurements, ultrasonography, and, especially, magnetic resonance imaging using metal artifact reduction sequence techniques to identify solid or fluid masses. These studies have identified increases in acetabular abduction angle, or "steeply inclined cups," as a cause of increased wear, sometimes with a dramatic increase in serum levels of cobalt and chromium[149]; the risk for high wear with steep implantation angle seems to be increased with small component sizes, especially in designs with a low coverage angle.[128,150–152]

ALTR I

Most modern metal-on-metal bearings have less volumetric wear and resultant osteolysis than was observed with systems containing conventional polyethylene components.[153] However, wear-particle related bone resorption with metal-on-metal bearings has been reported in a few publications,[154,155] including hip resurfacing.[156,157] Daniel and colleagues[158] reported a high rate of osteolysis and aseptic component loosening in a series of McMinn Devices (Corin Medical Ltd, Cirencester, UK) implanted in 1996. The investigators concluded that the heat treatment used with these devices was the cause of excessive wear, leading to an increased rate of loosening, compared with a group of patients who received similar devices with a different metallurgy process. However, this study failed to provide data on the clearance of the components used or any type of

in vivo wear measurement to substantiate their claim. This result is in contradiction with wear simulator studies,[159] even with bearings submitted to severe wear conditions.[160] Much of the current debate is to determine whether osteolysis is the result of a poorly functioning device with excessive wear production or the result of a patient's low threshold for reaction to metal-wear debris (ALTR III).[161] In a study by Amstutz and colleagues, 29 retrieved femoral resurfacing components were examined for wear. Four of those components were identified as ALTR I cases and 2 as ALTR II cases. Cases with ALTR had significantly higher linear wear rate, cup anteversion angle, and lower contact patch-to-rim distance than the other components (see the article by Amstutz and colleagues elsewhere in this issue for further exploration of this topic).

ALTR II

A high incidence (1.8%) of ALTR II reactions has recently been observed by a group of researchers from Oxford.[119] They reported higher linear femoral and acetabular wear rates for cases revised with pseudotumors compared with cases without.[162] Edge loading was observed in all acetabular components in the pseudotumor group. This publication did not describe the orientation of the socket in these cases. In contrast, another center with a large series of MMRA and comparable follow-up time reported a 0.15% prevalence of such reactions[123] and was able to provide explanations for the observed cases. The cause of ALTR II cases has been associated with the cytotoxicity of cobalt nanoparticles and seems to be dose dependent.[163] Revision surgery of ALTR II cases led to poor outcomes,[120] which suggests that all patients with metal-on-metal bearings should be regularly followed up and revised early after symptoms develop, before severe wear problems (osteolysis and muscle destruction) are detected. The investigators report a high incidence of dislocation after revision for ALTR II, but these revisions used 28- and 32-mm bearings rather than large or big femoral heads (BFH).[120]

ALTR III

The variable biologic reactivity of the patient is also a factor in the outcome of the surgery. There are several reports suggesting a high incidence of systemic allergy associated with a histologic diagnosis of aseptic lymphocyte-dominated vasculitis-associated lesion (ALVAL),[164,165] but wear analysis is rarely performed on these cases, which might in fact fall into the ALTR I or ALTR II category because of excessive wear. True allergic responses generally present within the first 2 years and are not necessarily associated with high wear.[126,127] There have been several case reports on ALTRs attributed to metal hypersensitivity. Molvik and colleagues[166] reported a case of groin mass associated with weight loss, night sweats, and increased levels of inflammatory markers in a 60-year-old woman with a metal-on-metal THR. Her acetabular component was found to be loose, along with 200 mL of purulent fluid in an inflammatory capsule and marked superior and anterior osteolysis. Histologic analysis revealed prominent perivascular infiltration of lymphocytes and plasma cells, along with macrophages with metal particles. In addition, Perumal and colleagues[167] also reported a case of soft tissue mass in a patient with metal-on-metal THR. This patient also had a loose acetabular component, and the soft tissue mass revealed metallic debris and lymphocytic infiltration, which they identified as delayed type IV cobalt hypersensitivity. Watters and colleagues[168] reported a case of pseudotumor with superimposed infection in a 75-year-old man with metal-on-metal THR. Tissue histology revealed metallic particles, with diffuse perivascular lymphocytic invasion with numerous plasma cells and multifocal acute inflammation with extensive fibrinous necrosis.

The term ALVAL was coined by Willert and colleagues[127] in a histologic study of tissues from metal-on-metal hips. At present, there is confusion and misuse of the term ALVAL; oftentimes, ALVAL is wrongly used as a diagnosis for metal sensitivity or used to describe a mode of failure. ALVAL is strictly a histologic term used to describe features associated with a delayed-type hypersensitivity-like reaction to metal particles, ions, and corrosion products in tissues from prosthetic joints. At this time, we are not aware of histologically verified cases with the Conserve® Plus in the United States, but several have been identified in Europe (see the article by De Smet and colleagues elsewhere in this issue for further exploration of this topic).

Prevention

Based on retrieval analyses,[30,42] it is clear that one of the major improvements in this era of metal-on-metal bearings is the reduction in wear provided by well-functioning modern-generation bearings. However, with some designs, and particularly when acetabular malpositioning resulted in steep cup angles (>55° of abduction), edge wear occurred,[169] producing much higher wear rates.[170]

De Haan and colleagues[150] showed the critical nature of the cup arc of cover, which varies with component positioning, size, and design. They reported higher ion levels with the BHR compared with the Conserve® Plus in hips with an abduction angle greater than 55 degrees. The coverage angle of the Conserve® Plus ranges from 159° to 164°, the BHR from 154° to 165°,[171] the ASR from 144° to 157°, and the Biomet Magnum (Biomet, Warsaw, IN, USA) from approximately 157° to 165° (estimates based on a figure from Griffin,[171] sizes 44–66). Even with a constant cover angle for all sizes, the cover area is reduced for small components compared with large components.[150] Therefore, a clear strategy to prevent wear-related failures is to optimize component orientation and coverage, that is, avoid excessive cup abduction angle or anteversion, especially in smaller sizes, and this becomes even more critical with the designs that present the lowest coverage angles (**Fig. 4**).

The knowledge regarding the tribology of metal-on-metal resurfaced joints continues to expand. New data suggest that wear may be reduced by as much as 50% by forging the harder femoral component and using it against the softer as-cast heat-treated and solution-annealed socket,[172] but this theory has not as yet been verified in vivo. Other new technologies suggest that there may be other ways of reducing wear, such as using a ceramic femoral component or ceramic coating or hardening the material.[173,174]

The most important preventive measure available at this time to minimize wear is to know the design characteristics and limitations of the components and orient the components in an optimal position. Guidelines for component orientation with respect to size were described for the ASR,[124] but because of poor coverage and a reported high incidence of ALTR, this device has been recalled from the US market. A safe zone needs to be identified for other designs as well, in relationship with component size. Manufacturers should take steps to optimize their socket design.

Systemic complications related to wear debris from metal-on-metal bearings have been mainly the subject of speculation this far because these effects, if they exist, take a long time to show clinical signs. Tharani and colleagues[175] reviewed the literature in an attempt to determine the carcinogenicity of THR and found no association but recognized the limitations of the data available in 2001. However, the recent report of 2 cases of cobaltism in patients with metal-on-metal stem-type THA has shown the possibility of reactions to metal debris beyond the tissues surrounding the prosthetic joint.[176] In his commentary related to this publication, Jacobs highlighted the rarity of this

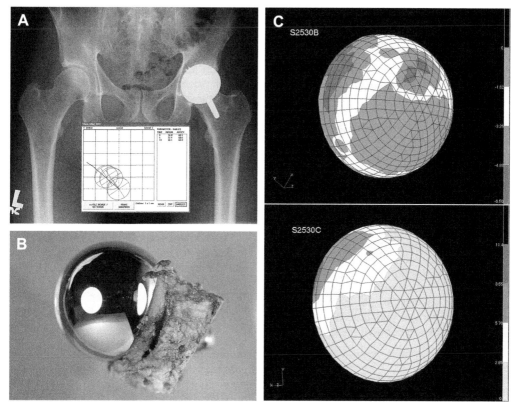

Fig. 4. (*A*) Anteroposterior radiograph of the pelvis of a 51-year-old man 1 year after BHR. Note the excessive anteversion angle of the acetabular component (>60°), which was confirmed by EBRA Cup studies (*inset*). (*B*) Retrieved femoral head with unique bone remodeling caused by impingement of the femoral neck with the acetabular component. (*C*) Wear measurements performed with coordinate measuring machine (CMM) on the retrieved components. Note the edge wear on both the acetabular and femoral components.

occurrence and pointed out that 4 of the 6 reported cases to date that have demonstrated chromium- and cobalt-associated neurologic and/or cardiac complications occurred with bearings other than metal-on-metal. His recommendations included a regular follow-up of patients with any kind of joint arthroplasty, including a discussion of the overall health of the patient, a blood or serum detection of metal levels in case of unexplained symptoms, and a prompt revision if evidence of high wear or corrosion lead to local or systemic complications.[177]

DISLOCATION AND IMPINGEMENT
Incidence and Significance

Dislocation occurs more rarely after hip resurfacing than after a traditional THA because the femoral head of the prosthesis is large and approximates the original femoral head size and the natural anatomy of the hip. The incidence of dislocation after MMRA usually ranges from 0% to 1%,[1,5,13,15,18,23,78,79,89,178–181] with 1 study

reporting 3.1%.[19] Even in groups of patients usually prone to this particular adverse event (eg, patients with hip dysplasia), hip resurfacing has shown excellent stability.[21,107–112,182,183] In comparison, dislocation is a common complication and cause for revision with conventional THR using traditional balls of sizes 28 and 32 mm.[184] However, the risk of dislocation (especially recurrent dislocation) is greatly reduced with a total hip prosthesis with a larger femoral head to prevent recurrent dislocation.[185,186]

Etiology

Although reported dislocation rates are usually low (<1%) with hip resurfacing, overall stability still depends on component positioning. If there is excessive anteversion, of either the femoral neck or the cup, anterior dislocation may occur. Posterior dislocation may occur as a result of impingement between the cup and the femoral neck. Impingement of the femoral neck and the acetabular component is a source of concern expressed by several publications on the range of motion provided by the resurfacing systems. Most of the publications that studied this issue used a computer model[187–189] or a physical construct[190] and outlined the theoretical concern of a smaller femoral component to neck diameter ratio in resurfacing compared with large-head THR. These results correlate with the findings of Ball and Schmalzried,[191] who reported on a series demonstrating radiographic signs of posterior impingement. Impingement may be a commonly occurring phenomenon that suggests that the optimal component positioning in resurfacing may present only a small margin for error. The clinical consequences of impingement seem to be of relatively minor importance[7] and mainly related to patients with supraphysiologic flexibility.[192] The clinically measured range-of-motion scores reported after resurfacing do not support this as being a concern.[193–195] There have been a few isolated reports of adverse effects, presumably as a result of impingement and possibly related to the use of a specific component design.[196]

Prevention

Component orientation, specifically with the acetabular component, plays a pivotal role in the clinical success of the resurfacing prosthesis. Many studies have highlighted the importance of component version[188] and lateral opening, suggesting that acetabular components placed in angles greater than 55° generate more wear than properly positioned components[149,150,157] because of edge loading. These figures should also be used as limits for risk of dislocation because edge loading constitutes the limit for the articular system before dislocation. Obtaining a precise positioning of the components can be challenging as shown by the learning curve experienced in most institutions. Despite this challenge, a few centers seem to have managed to successfully perform MMRA with a reduced incision length.[197–200] However, these techniques cannot be recommended for surgeons starting their resurfacing practice.[69]

Although impingement, in our experience, has not been associated with either symptoms or increased wear, we recommend that the position of the femoral component be optimally oriented to increase femoral head-neck offset, especially laterally and anteriorly to minimize the potential for impingement. This positioning is facilitated by an instrument system such as the Conserve® Plus, which permits changing the initial pin placement by means of a relocator guide for translation or angulation during the serial reaming process. Further fine-tuning is possible as the surgeon

approaches the final reaming by removing the pin, inserting the empty cylindrical reamer over the reamed bone, and reorienting either the varus-valgus direction or the anterior-posterior direction (go to orthopedic.theclinics.com to see author video). Then the pin can be reinserted to finish the reaming in the optimized direction for offset and to take advantage of the best bone for fixation, which becomes apparent during the reaming process. This is only possible when the stem hole is not drilled until that optimal position has been obtained.

HETEROTOPIC OSSIFICATION
Incidence and Significance

HO is seen after both THA and resurfacing hip arthroplasty in varying degrees. Following the classification system of Brooker and colleagues,[201] there are 4 degrees of ectopic bone formation: (1) grade I includes the initial formation of bone within the soft tissue about the hip, (2) grade II includes bone spurs from the pelvis or proximal end of the femur, with at least 1 cm between bone surfaces, (3) grade III includes bone spurs with less than 1 cm of space between opposing bone surfaces, and (4) grade IV is defined as apparent bone ankylosis. Grades I, II, and III are not considered to significantly alter the functional results as assessed by the Harris hip score.[201] The current literature reporting HO rates for modern resurfacing devices shows variable rates of incidence. Back and colleagues[202] reported an overall percentage of 58.6 with the BHR device, with 37.3% Brooker grade I, 13.18% Brooker grade II, and 8.2% Brooker grade III. In a series of 400 hips, HO was noted in 26.5% of the hips, with 28 hips (7%, all males) showing Brooker grade III or higher.[87] A randomized comparative study showed a higher incidence of severe HO (Brooker grades III and IV) in resurfacing than in THA, with rates of 12.6% and 2.1%, respectively.[203] These 3 studies are at the higher end of reported rates. Other centers have reported a more moderate incidence of severe HO ranging from 0% to 3.5%.[5,13,14,19,28,79,193] In an Asian population of patients, Nishii and colleagues[21] reported 1.5% overall and 1% grade III.

Although these results show a large variability, they are overall consistent with reports on HO after THA, which also show a wide range of incidence.[204–209]

Etiology

The cause is unknown, but men with osteoarthritis are at a greater risk of developing HO than other patient populations.[202] Muscle stretching and retained bone debris may also be risk factors specific to the resurfacing procedure.

Prevention

An effective prophylactic regimen has been described by Amstutz and colleagues,[68] in which all patients receive 100 mg of indomethacin suppository immediately after surgery and 25 mg 3 times a day for 5 days postoperatively. In an attempt to reduce the incidence of significant HO, 700 cGy of radiotherapy are administered 12 to 24 hours preoperatively in patients undergoing simultaneous bilateral procedures or in patients undergoing a second operation who have previously demonstrated formation of HO after a procedure on the contralateral hip (see **Fig. 4**). Muscle stretching can be minimized during the surgical phases that require moving the patient's leg and during acetabular preparation. Copious lavage with 4000 mL should suffice to remove all debris after cementation of the femoral component. A recent study showed the efficacy of a plastic drape used to collect bone debris during reaming of the femoral head.[210]

FEMORAL NERVE PALSY
Incidence and Etiology

The reported rates of nerve palsy after hip resurfacing are low, ranging from 0% to 1.6%.[1,12,22,178,179,211] Most reports highlight a greater risk of sequelae with sciatic or peroneal nerve palsies than with femoral nerve palsies. Usually, patients who suffer from damage (palsy) of the femoral nerve, which operates the quadriceps (knee extension), recover without residual effects. It is possible to injure the sciatic nerve much in the same way, and this potential complication can occur with a THR, but it is rare with the posterior approach (1 in 1000).[1]

To perform hip resurfacing, the surgeon must work around the femoral head to reach the acetabulum and implant the replacement in an optimal position. This procedure requires some additional stretching as compared with performing a conventional stem-type THR. Femoral neuropathies have been associated with the development of pseudotumors in 2 recent case reports.[121,212]

Prevention

Femoral nerve: it is recommended to release the capsule at the junction to the bone on the acetabulum and around the base of the neck. The time the femur is displaced anteriorly for socket preparation and implantation should be minimized so that the pressure on the femoral nerve is minimal. It is important to retract the posterior capsule posteriorly. A Charnley-type pin placed inside the capsule into the ischium is a helpful retractor.[68,70]

Sciatic nerve: Release if necessary the gluteus maximus linea aspera insertion with the electrocautery. The section of the quadratus femoris should be performed carefully. The release of the gluteal sling during a posterior approach, as well as flexing the knee during hip reduction, is thought to reduce the risk of sciatic nerve palsy during resurfacing.[213]

THROMBOEMBOLIC PHENOMENA
Incidence and Significance

All patients are at risk for blood clots following THR or resurfacing, but the rates do not differ between the 2 types of prosthetic devices.[24,28] Patel and colleagues[214] found no difference in cerebral microemboli between THA and resurfacing groups using transcranial Doppler ultrasonography. Many centers have reported the absence of deep vein thrombosis (DVT) in their resurfacing experience,[5,13,21,183] and the others have kept the incidence rate at less than 1%.[1,14,17,22,178] Patients undergoing hip resurfacing have been able to fly across the United States safely as early as 3 to 4 days after surgery.[215] These low rates of incidence are undoubtedly the result of effective prophylactic protocols used in all these centers as shown by a higher rate (10.4%) of DVT found in a study performed on 221 patients who underwent THA or MMRA without any thromboembolic prophylaxis.[216]

Prevention

Although the incidence of death is low following hip resurfacing, it is not zero. Chemical prophylaxis, combined with anti-embolism stockings and calf or other compression garments, is strongly recommended. Warfarin at a dose of 10 mg can be administered on the night of surgery and subsequently for 3 weeks, with a dose adjusted to maintain the international normalized ratio between 1.8 and 2.5. Aspirin is then given for an additional 3 weeks.[68,70] This regimen can generally be monitored by internal medicine physicians. Injectable heparins are also efficacious, but their safety has been questioned with a higher incidence of wound complications, although comparative controlled studies have not been performed with hip resurfacing. The use of intermittent pneumatic calf compression has shown efficacy in reducing the incidence of thromboembolic events.[217]

DISCUSSION

Despite the rebirth of hip resurfacing with metal-on-metal bearings being a success, complications still exist, some of them specific to this type of procedure. Our purpose was to investigate the incidence rates of these particular complications, their causes, and the techniques to reduce these incidence rates through a search of the peer-reviewed literature.

A limitation of the systematic review process in the study of complications after MMRA was that clinical articles usually list the complications that occurred during the study in the body of the text, without a specific mention in the abstract. For this reason, many studies providing this information had to be added to the review after the systematic computerized search. A keyword search of the full-text (Adobe) documents and the investigators' previous knowledge of the related literature proved essential for our purpose. For the particular topics addressed in the present review, up to 40 articles had to be added this way for a particular section.

The main finding from this review was that all complication rates were low overall, confirming the safety and efficacy of the procedure. Also, we found that the variability in the incidence of complications was usually greater between centers than between designs or between patient populations. This finding tends to show that surgical technique is likely to be the most important factor toward a reduction of complication rates. Surgeons who take up this technique need to be students of all of the experiences recorded, including books on hip resurfacing and the published peer-reviewed literature, especially in the last 2 years. Because of a known learning curve,[22,218,219] surgeons who are not experienced with resurfacing arthroplasty and are not students of the technique should not take on challenging cases, such as patients with several large femoral cysts and small components, especially in combination with a low BMI. A smaller head is a risk factor in both the male and female cohorts, most likely because of a reduced surface area for fixation, thus affecting the initial fixation. However, the strong effect of surgical technique improvements over time suggests that even individuals with a small head can benefit from resurfacing performed in a center with a large experience using optimal technique with the procedure.[1,19,97] This especially benefits women, who have a greater percentage of small component sizes. However, recently it is becoming more apparent that component orientation is critical to minimize wear by edge loading, an adverse effect that is design related and more apparent with small component sizes.

SUMMARY

The goals of resurfacing are to be conserving bone for the acetabulum and the femur, restoring anatomy and biomechanics with equal leg lengths, and providing dislocation-free function and the ability to revise simply. It is anticipated that results will continue to improve by reducing complications and failures.

SUPPLEMENTARY DATA

Supplementary data related to this article can be found online at doi:10.1016/j.ocl.2010.12.002.

REFERENCES

1. Amstutz H, Le Duff M. Eleven years of experience with metal-on-metal hybrid hip resurfacing: a review of 1000 Conserve Plus. J Arthroplasty 2008;23(6 Suppl 1):36–43.
2. Bohm R, Schraml A, Schuh A. Long-term results with the Wagner metal-on-metal hip resurfacing prosthesis. Hip Int 2006;16(2):58–64.
3. McMinn D, Treacy R, Lin K, et al. Metal on metal surface replacement of the hip. Experience of the McMinn prothesis. Clin Orthop Relat Res 1996; 329(Suppl):S89–98.
4. Shimmin A, Beaulé PE, Campbell P. Metal-on-metal hip resurfacing arthroplasty. J Bone Joint Surg Am 2008;90(3):637–54.
5. Treacy R, McBryde C, Pynsent P. Birmingham hip resurfacing arthroplasty. A minimum follow-up of five years. J Bone Joint Surg Br 2005;87(2):167–70.
6. Wagner M, Wagner H. Preliminary results of uncemented metal on metal stemmed and resurfacing hip replacement arthroplasty. Clin Orthop Relat Res 1996;329(Suppl):S78–88.
7. Amstutz H, Le Duff M, Campbell P, et al. Clinical and radiographic results of metal-on-metal hip resurfacing with a minimum ten-year follow-up. J Bone Joint Surg Am 2010;92(16):2663–71.
8. Howie DW, Campbell D, McGee M, et al. Wagner resurfacing hip arthroplasty. The results of one hundred consecutive arthroplasties after eight to ten years. J Bone Joint Surg Am 1990;72(5):708–14.
9. Sahlgrenska University Hospital Department of Orthopaedics. The Swedish National Hip Arthroplasty Register–Annual report. 2008. p. 59. Available at: www.jru.orthop.gu.se. Accessed December 20, 2010.
10. Beaulé P, Shim P, Banga K. Clinical experience of Ganz surgical dislocation approach for metal-on-metal hip resurfacing. J Arthroplasty 2009; 24(Suppl 6):127–31.

11. Cutts S, Datta A, Ayoub K, et al. Early failure modalities in hip resurfacing. Hip Int 2005;15:155–8.

12. Della Valle C, Nunley R, Raterman S, et al. Initial American experience with hip resurfacing following FDA approval. Clin Orthop Relat Res 2008;467(1):72–8.

13. Heilpern G, Shah N, Fordyce M. Birmingham hip resurfacing arthroplasty: a series of 110 consecutive hips with a minimum five-year clinical and radiological follow-up. J Bone Joint Surg Br 2008;90(9):1137–42.

14. Jameson S, Langton D, Nargol A. Articular surface replacement of the hip: a prospective single-surgeon series. J Bone Joint Surg Br 2010;92(1):28–37.

15. Khan M, Kuiper J, Edwards D, et al. Birmingham hip arthroplasty five to eight years of prospective multi-center results. J Arthroplasty 2009;24(7):1044–50.

16. Kim P, Beaulé P, Laflamme G, et al. Causes of early failure in a multicenter clinical trial of hip resurfacing. J Arthroplasty 2008;23(6 Suppl 1):44–9.

17. Madhu T, Akula M, Raman R, et al. The Birmingham hip resurfacing prosthesis: an independent single surgeon's experience at 7-year follow-up. J Arthroplasty 2011;26(1):1–8.

18. McAndrew A, Khaleel A, Bloomfield M, et al. A district general hospital's experience of hip resurfacing. Hip Int 2007;17(1):1–3.

19. Mont M, Seyler T, Ulrich S, et al. Effect of changing indications and techniques on total hip resurfacing. Clin Orthop Relat Res 2007;465:63–70.

20. Marker D, Seyler T, Jinnah R, et al. Femoral neck fractures after metal-on-metal total hip resurfacing: a prospective cohort study. J Arthroplasty 2007;22(7 Suppl 3):66–71.

21. Nishii T, Sugano N, Miki H, et al. Five-year results of metal-on-metal resurfacing arthroplasty in Asian patients. J Arthroplasty 2007;22(2):176–83.

22. O'Neill M, Beaule P, Bin Nasser A, et al. Canadian academic experience with metal-on-metal hip resurfacing. Bull NYU Hosp Jt Dis 2009;67(2):128–31.

23. Ollivere B, Duckett S, August A, et al. The Birmingham hip resurfacing: 5-year clinical and radiographic results from a district general hospital. Int Orthop 2010;34(5):631–4.

24. Pollard T, Baker R, Eastaugh-Waring S, et al. Treatment of the young active patient with osteoarthritis of the hip. A five- to seven-year comparison of hybrid total hip arthroplasty and metal-on-metal resurfacing. J Bone Joint Surg Br 2006;88(5):592–600.

25. Shimmin A, Back D. Femoral neck fractures following Birmingham hip resurfacing. J Bone Joint Surg Br 2005;87(4):463–4.

26. Siebel T, Maubach S, Morlock M. Lessons learned from early clinical experience and results of 300 ASR hip resurfacing implantations. Proc Inst Mech Eng H 2006;220(2):345–53.

27. Steffen R, Foguet P, Krikler S, et al. Femoral neck fractures after hip resurfacing. J Arthroplasty 2009;24(4):614–9.

28. Vail T, Mina C, Yergler J, et al. Metal-on-metal hip resurfacing compares favorably with THA at 2 years follow-up. Clin Orthop Relat Res 2006;453:123–31.

29. Witzleb W, Arnold M, Krummenauer F, et al. Birmingham hip resurfacing arthroplasty: short-term clinical and radiographic outcome. Eur J Med Res 2008;13(1):39–46.

30. Campbell P, Beaulé P, Ebramzadeh E, et al. A study of implant failure in metal-on-metal surface arthroplasties. Clin Orthop 2006;453:35–46.

31. Ganapathi M, Evans S, Roberts P. Strain pattern following surface replacement of the hip. Proc Inst Mech Eng H 2008;222(1):13–8.

32. Long J, Santner T, Bartel D. Hip resurfacing increases bone strains associated with short-term femoral neck fracture. J Orthop Res 2009;27(10):1319–25.

33. Taylor M. Finite element analysis of the resurfaced femoral head. Proc Inst Mech Eng H 2006;220(2):289–97.

34. Anglin C, Masri B, Tonetti J, et al. Hip resurfacing femoral neck fracture influenced by valgus placement. Clin Orthop Relat Res 2007;465:71–9.

35. Radcliffe I, Taylor M. Investigation into the effect of varus-valgus orientation on load transfer in the resurfaced femoral head: a multi-femur finite element analysis. Clin Biomech 2007;22(7):780–6.

36. Richards C, Giannitsios D, Huk O, et al. Risk of periprosthetic femoral neck fracture after hip resurfacing arthroplasty: valgus compared with anatomic alignment. A biomechanical and clinical analysis. J Bone Joint Surg Am 2008;90(Suppl 3):96–101.

37. Davis E, Olsen M, Zdero R, et al. Femoral neck fracture following hip resurfacing: the effect of alignment of the femoral component. J Bone Joint Surg Br 2008;90(11):1522–7.

38. Vail T, Glisson R, Dominguez D, et al. Position of hip resurfacing component affects strain and resistance to fracture in the femoral neck. J Bone Joint Surg Am 2008;90(9):1951–60.

39. Amstutz H, Campbell P, Le Duff M. Fracture of the neck of the femur after surface arthroplasty of the hip. J Bone Joint Surg Am 2004;86(9):1874–7.

40. Cossey A, Back D, Shimmin A, et al. The non-operative management of periprosthetic fractures associated with the Birmingham hip resurfacing procedure. J Arthroplasty 2005;20(3):358–61.

41. Campbell P, Takamura K, Lundergan W, et al. Cement technique changes improved hip resurfacing longevity: implant retrieval findings. Bull NYU Hosp Jt Dis 2009;67(2):146–53.

42. Morlock M, Bishop N, Zustin J, et al. Modes of implant failure after hip resurfacing: morphological

and wear analysis of 267 retrieval specimens. J Bone Joint Surg Am 2008;90(Suppl 3):89–95.

43. Schlegel U, Knifka J, Röllinghoff M, et al. Effects of impaction on cement mantle and trabecular bone in hip resurfacing. Arch Orthop Trauma Surg 2010. [Epub ahead of print].

44. Schlegel U, Rothstock S, Siewe J, et al. Does impaction matter in hip resurfacing? A cadaveric study. J Arthroplasty 2011;26(2):296–302.

45. Little J, Gray H, Murray D, et al. Thermal effects of cement mantle thickness for hip resurfacing. J Arthroplasty 2008;23(3):454–8.

46. Gill H, Campbell P, Murray D, et al. Reduction of the potential for thermal damage during hip resurfacing. J Bone Joint Surg Br 2007;89(1):16–20.

47. Bitsch R, Heisel C, Silva M, et al. Femoral cementing technique for hip resurfacing arthroplasty. J Orthop Res 2007;25(4):423–31.

48. Bitsch R, Loidolt T, Heisel C, et al. Cementing techniques for hip resurfacing arthroplasty: in vitro study of pressure and temperature. J Arthroplasty 2011;26(1):144–51.

49. Little C, Ruiz A, Harding I, et al. Osteonecrosis in retrieved femoral heads after failed resurfacing arthroplasty of the hip. J Bone Joint Surg Br 2005; 87(3):320–3.

50. Steffen R, Fern D, Norton M, et al. Femoral oxygenation during hip resurfacing through the trochanteric flip approach. Clin Orthop Relat Res 2009; 467(4):934–9.

51. Amarasekera H, Costa M, Foguet P, et al. The blood flow to the femoral head/neck junction during resurfacing arthroplasty: a comparison of two approaches using laser Doppler flowmetry. J Bone Joint Surg Br 2008;90(4):442–5.

52. Beaulé P, Campbell P, Hoke R, et al. Notching of the femoral neck during resurfacing arthroplasty of the hip: a vascular study. J Bone Joint Surg Br 2006;88(6):35–9.

53. Beaulé P, Campbell P, Shim P. Femoral head blood flow during hip resurfacing. Clin Orthop Relat Res 2007;456:148–52.

54. Khan A, Yates P, Lovering A, et al. The effect of surgical approach on blood flow to the femoral head during resurfacing. J Bone Joint Surg Br 2007;89(1):21–5.

55. Forrest N, Welch A, Murray A, et al. Femoral head viability after Birmingham resurfacing hip arthroplasty: assessment with use of [18F] fluoride positron emission tomography. J Bone Joint Surg Am 2006;88(Suppl 3):84–9.

56. Ullmark G, Sundgren K, Milbrink J, et al. Osteonecrosis following resurfacing arthroplasty. Acta Orthop 2009;80(6):670–4.

57. Hananouchi T, Nishii T, Lee S, et al. The vascular network in the femoral head and neck after hip resurfacing. J Arthroplasty 2010;25(1):146–51.

58. Harty J, Devitt B, Harty L, et al. Dual energy x-ray absorptiometry analysis of peri-prosthetic stress shielding in the Birmingham resurfacing hip replacement. Arch Orthop Trauma Surg 2005;125(10):693–5.

59. Hayaishi Y, Miki H, Nishii T, et al. Proximal femoral bone mineral density after resurfacing total hip arthroplasty and after standard stem-type cementless total hip arthroplasty, both having similar neck preservation and the same articulation type. J Arthroplasty 2007;22(8):1208–13.

60. Amstutz H, Ball S, Le Duff M, et al. Hip resurfacing for patients under 50 years of age. Results of 350 Conserve Plus with a 2–9 year follow-up. Clin Orthop Relat Res 2007;460:159–64.

61. McGrath M, Desser D, Ulrich S, et al. Total hip resurfacing in patients who are sixty years of age or older. J Bone Joint Surg Am 2008;90(Suppl 3): 27–31.

62. The North American Menopause Society. Serious health issues at menopause. Menopause. vol. 2009. Mayfield Heights (OH): Lippincott Williams & Wilkins; 2009.

63. Ahlborg H, Johnell O, Turner C, et al. Bone loss and bone size after menopause. N Engl J Med 2003; 349(4):327–34.

64. Arden NK, Griffiths GO, Hart DJ, et al. The association between osteoarthritis and osteoporotic fracture: the Chingford Study. Br J Rheumatol 1996; 35(12):1299–304.

65. Cumming R, Klineberg R. Epidemiological study of the relation between arthritis of the hip and hip fractures. Ann Rheum Dis 1993;52:707–10.

66. Dequeker J, Johnell O. Osteoarthritis protects against femoral neck fracture: the MEDOS study experience. Bone 1993;14(Suppl 1):S51–6.

67. Foss M, Byers P. Bone density, osteoarthrosis of the hip, and fracture of the upper end of the femur. Ann Rheum Dis 1972;31:259–64.

68. Amstutz H, Beaulé P, Dorey F, et al. Metal-on-metal hybrid surface arthroplasty – surgical technique. J Bone Joint Surg Am 2006;88(Suppl 1 Pt 2): 234–49.

69. Amstutz H. "Top 10" technical pearls for successfully performing hip resurfacing arthroplasty. Tech Orthop 2010;25(1):73–9.

70. Amstutz H. Surgical technique. In: Amstutz HC, editor. Hip resurfacing: principles, indications, technique and results. Philadelphia: Elsevier; 2008. p. 77–94.

71. Benoit B, Gofton W, Beaulé P. Hueter anterior approach for hip resurfacing: assessment of the learning curve. Orthop Clin North Am 2009;40(3): 357–63.

72. Nork S, Schär M, Pfander G, et al. Anatomic considerations for the choice of surgical approach for hip resurfacing arthroplasty. Orthop Clin North Am 2005;36(2):163–70.

73. Sandri A, Regis D, Magnan B, et al. Hip resurfacing using the anterolateral Watson-Jones approach in the supine position. Orthopedics 2009;32(6):406.

74. Bailey C, Gul R, Falworth M, et al. Component alignment in hip resurfacing using computer navigation. Clin Orthop Relat Res 2009;467(4):917–22.

75. Hodgson A, Helmy N, Masri B, et al. Comparative repeatability of guide-pin axis positioning in computer-assisted and manual femoral head resurfacing arthroplasty. Proc Inst Mech Eng H 2007; 221(7):713–24.

76. Pal B, Gupta S, New A. A numerical study of failure mechanisms in the cemented resurfaced femur: effects of interface characteristics and bone remodelling. Proc Inst Mech Eng H 2009;223(4):471–84.

77. Gupta S, New A, Taylor M. Bone remodelling inside a cemented resurfaced femoral head. Clin Biomech 2006;21(6):594–602.

78. Hing C, Back D, Bailey M, et al. The results of primary Birmingham hip resurfacings at a mean of five years. An independent prospective review of the first 230 hips. J Bone Joint Surg Br 2007; 89(11):1431–8.

79. Steffen R, Pandit H, Palan J, et al. The five-year results of the Birmingham hip resurfacing arthroplasty: an independent series. J Bone Joint Surg Br 2008;90(4):436–41.

80. McMinn D, Daniel J, Pradhan C, et al. Avascular necrosis in the young patient: a trilogy of arthroplasty options. Orthopedics 2005;28(9):945–7.

81. Revell M, McBryde C, Bhatnagar S, et al. Metal-on-metal hip resurfacing in osteonecrosis of the femoral head. J Bone Joint Surg Am 2006; 88(Suppl 3):98–103.

82. Mont M, Seyler T, Marker D, et al. Use of metal-on-metal total hip resurfacing for the treatment of osteonecrosis of the femoral head. J Bone Joint Surg Am 2006;88(Suppl 3):90–7.

83. Amstutz H, Le Duff M. Hip resurfacing results for osteonecrosis are as good as for other etiologies at 2 to 12 years. Clin Orthop Relat Res 2010; 468(2):375–81.

84. Beaulé P, Amstutz H, Le Duff M, et al. Surface arthroplasty for osteonecrosis of the hip: hemiresurfacing versus metal-on-metal hybrid resurfacing. J Arthroplasty 2004;19(12):54–8.

85. Gross T, Back F. Metal-on-metal hip resurfacing with an uncemented femoral component. A seven-year follow-up study. J Bone Joint Surg Am 2008;90(Suppl 3):32–7.

86. Lilikakis A, Vowler S, Villar R. Hydroxyapatite-coated femoral implant in metal-on-metal resurfacing hip arthroplasty: minimum of two years follow-up. Orthop Clin North Am 2005;36(2):215–22.

87. Amstutz H, Beaulé P, Dorey F, et al. Metal-on-metal hybrid surface arthroplasty: two to six year follow-up. J Bone Joint Surg Am 2004;86:28–39.

88. Le Duff M, Amstutz H, Dorey F. Metal-on-metal hip resurfacing for obese patients. J Bone Joint Surg Am 2007;89(12):2705–11.

89. Ramakrishnan R, Jaffe W, Kennedy WR. Metal-on-metal hip resurfacing radiographic evaluation techniques. J Arthroplasty 2008;23(8):1099–104.

90. Beaulé P, Krismer M, Mayrhofer P, et al. EBRA-FCA for measurement of migration of the femoral component in surface arthroplasty of the hip. J Bone Joint Surg Br 2005;87(5):741–4.

91. Itayem R, Arndt A, McMinn D, et al. A five-year radiostereometric follow-up of the Birmingham hip resurfacing arthroplasty. J Bone Joint Surg Br 2007;89(9):1140–3.

92. Falez F, Favetti F, Casella F, et al. Hip resurfacing: why does it fail? Early results and critical analysis of our first 60 cases. Int Orthop 2008;32(2):209–16.

93. Watanabe Y, Shiba N, Matsuo S, et al. Biomechanical study of the resurfacing hip arthroplasty: finite element analysis of the femoral component. J Arthroplasty 2000;15(4):505–11.

94. Long J, Bartel D. Surgical variables affect the mechanics of a hip resurfacing system. Clin Orthop Relat Res 2006;453:115–22.

95. Ong K, Day J, Kurtz S, et al. Role of surgical position on interface stress and initial bone remodeling stimulus around hip resurfacing arthroplasty. J Arthroplasty 2008;24(7):1137–42.

96. Schreiber A, Jacob H. Loosening of the femoral component of the ICLH double cup hip prosthesis. A biomechanical investigation with reference to clinical results. Acta Orthop Scand Suppl 1984; 207:1–34.

97. Amstutz H, Le Duff M, Campbell P, et al. The effects of technique changes on aseptic loosening of the femoral component in hip resurfacing. Results of 600 Conserve Plus with a 3–9 year follow-up. J Arthroplasty 2007;22(4):481–9.

98. Beaulé P, Matar WY, Poitras P, et al. 2008 Otto Aufranc Award: component design and technique affect cement penetration in hip resurfacing. Clin Orthop 2008;467(1):84–93.

99. Amstutz H, Le Duff M. Cementing the metaphyseal stem in metal-on-metal resurfacing: when and why. Clin Orthop Relat Res 2009;467(1):79–83.

100. Radcliffe I, Taylor M. Investigation into the affect of cementing techniques on load transfer in the resurfaced femoral head: a multi-femur finite element analysis. Clin Biomech (Bristol, Avon) 2007;22(4): 422–30.

101. Beaulé P, Le Duff M, Campbell P, et al. Metal-on-metal surface arthroplasty with a cemented femoral component: a 7–10 year follow-up study. J Arthroplasty 2004;19(12):17–22.

102. Dixon S, Jeavons L, Reddy R, et al. Early failure of the Dual coat Cormet 2000 metal on metal acetabular component. Hip Int 2009;19(2):128–30.

103. Long W, Dastane M, Harris M, et al. Failure of the Durom Metasul acetabular component. Clin Orthop Relat Res 2010;468(2):400–5.

104. Lavigne M, Therrien M, Nantel J, et al. The John Charnley Award: the functional outcome of hip resurfacing and large-head THA is the same: a randomized, double-blind study. Clin Orthop Relat Res 2010;468(2):326–36.

105. Vendittoli P, Lavigne M, Roy A, et al. A prospective randomized clinical trial comparing metal-on-metal total hip arthroplasty and metal-on-metal total hip resurfacing in patients less than 65 years old. Hip Int 2006;16(Suppl 4):873–81.

106. Davlin LB, Amstutz HC, Tooke SM, et al. Treatment of osteoarthrosis secondary to congenital dislocation of the hip. Primary cemented surface replacement compared with conventional total hip replacement. J Bone Joint Surg Am 1990;72(7):1035–42.

107. Naal F, Schmied M, Munzinger U, et al. Outcome of hip resurfacing arthroplasty in patients with developmental hip dysplasia. Clin Orthop Relat Res 2008;467:1516–21.

108. Xu W, Li J, Zhou Z, et al. Results of hip resurfacing for developmental dysplasia of the hip of Crowe type I and II. Chin Med J (Engl) 2008;121(15):1379–83.

109. McMinn D, Daniel J, Ziaee H, et al. Results of the Birmingham hip resurfacing dysplasia component in severe acetabular insufficiency: a six- to 9.6-year follow-up. J Bone Joint Surg Br 2008;90(6):715–23.

110. Amstutz H, Antoniades J, Le Duff M. Results of metal-on-metal hybrid hip resurfacing for Crowe type I and II developmental dysplasia. J Bone Joint Surg Am 2007;89(2):339–46.

111. Amstutz H, Le Duff M, Harvey N, et al. Improved survivorship of hybrid metal-on-metal hip resurfacing with second-generation techniques for Crowe I and II developmental dysplasia of the hip. J Bone Joint Surg 2008;90(Suppl 3):12–20.

112. McBryde C, Shears E, O'Hara J, et al. Metal-on-metal hip resurfacing in developmental dysplasia: a case-control study. J Bone Joint Surg Br 2008;90(6):708–14.

113. Schmalzried T. Metal-metal bearing surfaces in hip arthroplasty. Orthopedics 2009;32(9). DOI:10.3928/01477447-20090728-06. Available at: http://www.orthosupersite.com/view.asp?rID=42831. Accessed December 20, 2010.

114. Daniel J, Ziaee H, Pynsent P, et al. The validity of serum levels as a surrogate measure of systemic exposure to metal ions in hip replacement. J Bone Joint Surg Br 2007;89(6):736–41.

115. Walter L, Marel E, Harbury R, et al. Distribution of chromium and cobalt ions in various blood fractions after resurfacing hip arthroplasty. J Arthroplasty 2008;23(6):814–21.

116. Khan M, Takahashi T, Kuiper J, et al. Current in vivo wear of metal-on-metal bearings assessed by exercise-related rise in plasma cobalt level. J Orthop Res 2006;24(11):2029–35.

117. Khan M, Kuiper J, Richardson J. The exercise-related rise in plasma cobalt levels after metal-on-metal hip resurfacing arthroplasty. J Bone Joint Surg Br 2008;90(9):1152–7.

118. Pandit H, Glyn-Jones S, McLardy-Smith P, et al. Pseudotumours associated with metal-on-metal hip resurfacings. J Bone Joint Surg Br 2008;90(7):847–51.

119. Glyn-Jones S, Pandit H, Kwon Y, et al. Risk factors for inflammatory pseudotumour formation following hip resurfacing. J Bone Joint Surg Br 2009;91(12):1566–74.

120. Grammatopoulos G, Pandit H, Kwon Y, et al. Hip resurfacings revised for inflammatory pseudotumour have a poor outcome. J Bone Joint Surg Br 2009;91(8):1019–24.

121. Harvie P, Giele H, Fang C, et al. The treatment of femoral neuropathy due to pseudotumour caused by metal-on-metal resurfacing arthroplasty. Hip Int 2008;18(4):313–20.

122. Kwon Y, Ostlere S, McLardy-Smith P, et al. "Asymptomatic" pseudotumors after metal-on-metal hip resurfacing arthroplasty prevalence and metal ion study. J Arthroplasty 2010. [Epub ahead of print].

123. Malviya A, Holland J. Pseudotumours associated with metal-on-metal hip resurfacing: 10-year Newcastle experience. Acta Orthop Belg 2009;75(4):477–84.

124. Langton D, Jameson S, Joyce T, et al. Early failure of metal-on-metal bearings in hip resurfacing and large-diameter total hip replacement: a consequence of excess wear. J Bone Joint Surg Br 2010;92(1):38–46.

125. Mahendra G, Pandit H, Kliskey K, et al. Necrotic and inflammatory changes in metal-on-metal resurfacing hip arthroplasties. Acta Orthop 2009;80(6):653–9.

126. Campbell P, Shimmin A, Walter L, et al. Metal sensitivity as a cause of groin pain in metal-on-metal hip resurfacing. J Arthroplasty 2008;23(7):1080–5.

127. Willert H, Buchhorn G, Fayyazi A, et al. Metal-on-metal bearings and hypersensitivity in patients with artificial hip joints. A clinical and histomorphological study. J Bone Joint Surg Am 2005;87(1):28–36.

128. Ollivere B, Darrah C, Barker T, et al. Early clinical failure of the Birmingham metal-on-metal hip resurfacing is associated with metallosis and soft-tissue necrosis. J Bone Joint Surg Br 2009;91(8):1025–30.

129. Dowson D, Hardaker C, Flett M, et al. A hip joint simulator study of the performance of metal-on-metal joints. Part I. the role of materials. J Arthroplasty 2004;19(8 Suppl 3):118–23.

130. Dowson D, Hardaker C, Flett M, et al. A hip joint simulator study of the performance of metal-on-

metal joints. Part II. Design. J Arthroplasty 2004; 19(8 Suppl 3):124–30.

131. Rieker C, Schon R, Konrad R, et al. Influence of the clearance on in-vitro tribology of large diameter metal-on-metal articulations pertaining to resurfacing hip implants. Orthop Clin North Am 2005;36(2): 135–42.

132. Leslie I, Williams S, Brown C, et al. Effect of bearing size on the long-term wear, wear debris, and ion levels of large diameter metal-on-metal hip replacements—an in vitro study. J Biomed Mater Res B Appl Biomater 2008;87(1):163–72.

133. Vassiliou K, Elfick A, Scholes S, et al. The effect of 'running-in' on the tribology and surface morphology of metal-on-metal Birmingham hip resurfacing device in simulator studies. Proc Inst Mech Eng H 2006;220(2):269–77.

134. Wimmer M, Fischer A, Büscher R, et al. Wear mechanisms in metal-on-metal bearings: the importance of tribochemical reaction layers. J Orthop Res 2010;28(4):436–43.

135. Clarke M, Lee P, Arora A, et al. Levels of metal ions after small and large diameter metal-on-metal hip arthroplasty. J Bone Joint Surg Br 2003;85(6):913–7.

136. Daniel J, Ziaee H, Salama A, et al. The effect of the diameter of metal-on-metal bearings on systemic exposure to cobalt and chromium. J Bone Joint Surg Br 2006;88(4):443–8.

137. Moroni A, Savarino L, Cadossi M, et al. Does ion release differ between hip resurfacing and metal-on-metal THA? Clin Orthop Relat Res 2008; 466(3):700–7.

138. Vendittoli P, Roy A, Mottard S, et al. Metal ion release from bearing wear and corrosion with 28 mm and large-diameter metal-on-metal bearing articulations: a follow-up study. J Bone Joint Surg Br 2010;92(1):12–9.

139. Daniel J, Ziaee H, Pradhan C, et al. Blood and urine metal ion levels in young and active patients after Birmingham hip resurfacing arthroplasty: four-year results of a prospective longitudinal study. J Bone Joint Surg Br 2007;89(2):169–73.

140. Daniel J, Ziaee H, Pradhan C, et al. Six-year results of a prospective study of metal ion levels in young patients with metal-on-metal hip resurfacings. J Bone Joint Surg Br 2009;91(2):176–9.

141. Heisel C, Streich N, Krachler M, et al. Characterization of the running-in period in total hip resurfacing arthroplasty: an in vivo and in vitro metal ion analysis. J Bone Joint Surg Am 2008;90(Suppl 3): 125–33.

142. Hardaker C, Dowson D, Isaac G. Head replacement, head rotation, and surface damage effects of metal-on-metal total hip replacements: a hip simulator study. Proc Inst Mech Eng H 2004; 220(2):209–17.

143. Lee R, Essner A, Wang A. Tribological considerations in primary and revision metal-on-metal arthroplasty. J Bone Joint Surg Am 2008;90(Suppl 3):118–24.

144. Catelas I, Medley J, Campbell P, et al. Comparison of in vitro with in vivo characteristics of wear particles from metal-metal hip implants. J Biomed Mater Res B Appl Biomater 2004;70(2):167–78.

145. Doorn PF, Campbell PA, Worrall J, et al. Metal wear particle characterization from metal on metal total hip replacements: transmission electron microscopy study of periprosthetic tissues and isolated particles. J Biomed Mater Res 1998;42(1):103–11.

146. Jacobs J, Urban R, Hallab N, et al. Metal-on-metal bearing surfaces. J Am Acad Orthop Surg 2009; 17(2):69–76.

147. Davies A, Willert H, Campbell P, et al. An unusual lymphocytic perivascular infiltration in tissues around contemporary metal-on-metal joint replacements. J Bone Joint Surg Am 2005;87(1):18–27.

148. Langton D, Sprowson A, Mahadeva D, et al. Cup anteversion in hip resurfacing: validation of EBRA and the presentation of a simple clinical grading system. J Arthroplasty 2009;25(4):607–13.

149. Hart A, Buddhdev P, Winship P, et al. Cup inclination angle of greater than 50 degrees increases whole blood concentrations of cobalt and chromium ions after metal-on-metal hip resurfacing. Hip Int 2008;18(3):212–9.

150. De Haan R, Pattyn C, Gill H, et al. Correlation between inclination of the acetabular component and metal ion levels in metal-on-metal hip resurfacing replacement. J Bone Joint Surg Br 2008;90(10): 1291–7.

151. Langton D, Jameson S, Joyce T, et al. The effect of component size and orientation on the concentrations of metal ions after resurfacing arthroplasty of the hip. J Bone Joint Surg Br 2008;90(9):1143–51.

152. Vendittoli P, Mottard S, Roy A, et al. Chromium and cobalt ion release following the Durom high carbon content, forged metal-on-metal surface replacement of the hip. J Bone Joint Surg Br 2007;89(4): 441–8.

153. Callaghan J, Cuckler J, Huddleston J, et al. How have alternative bearings (such as metal-on-metal, highly cross-linked polyethylene, and ceramic-on-ceramic) affected the prevention and treatment of osteolysis? J Am Acad Orthop Surg 2008;16(Suppl 1):S33–8.

154. Korovessis P, Petsinis G, Repanti M, et al. Metallosis after contemporary metal-on-metal total hip arthroplasty. Five to nine-year follow-up. J Bone Joint Surg Am 2006;88(6):1183–91.

155. Park Y, Moon Y, Lim S, et al. Early osteolysis following second-generation metal-on-metal hip replacement. J Bone Joint Surg Am 2005;87(7): 1515–21.

156. Costi K, Howie D, Campbell D, et al. Long-term survival and reason for revision of Wagner resurfacing hip arthroplasty. J Arthroplasty 2010;25(4):522–8.

157. De Haan R, Campbell P, Su E, et al. Revision of metal-on-metal resurfacing arthroplasty of the hip: the influence of malpositioning of the components. J Bone Joint Surg Br 2008;90(9):1158–63.

158. Daniel J, Ziaee H, Kamali A, et al. Ten-year results of a double-heat-treated metal-on-metal hip resurfacing. J Bone Joint Surg Br 2010;92(1):20–7.

159. Nevelos J, Shelton J, Fisher J. Metallurgical considerations in the wear of metal-on-metal hip bearings. Hip Int 2004;14(1):1–10.

160. Bowsher J, Nevelos J, Williams P, et al. 'Severe' wear challenge to 'as-cast' and 'double heat-treated' large-diameter metal-on-metal hip bearings. Proc Inst Mech Eng H 2006;220(2):135–43.

161. Carr A, DeSteiger R. Osteolysis in patients with a metal-on-metal hip arthroplasty. ANZ J Surg 2008;78(3):144–7.

162. Kwon Y, Glyn-Jones S, Simpson DJ, et al. Analysis of wear of retrieved metal-on-metal hip resurfacing implants revised due to pseudotumors. J Bone Joint Surg Br 2010;92(3):356–61.

163. Kwon Y, Xia Z, Glyn-Jones S, et al. Dose-dependent cytotoxicity of clinically relevant cobalt nanoparticles and ions on macrophages in vitro. Biomed Mater 2009;4(2):25018.

164. Zustin J, Amling M, Krause M, et al. Intraosseous lymphocytic infiltrates after hip resurfacing arthroplasty: a histopathological study on 181 retrieved femoral remnants. Virchows Arch 2009;454(5): 581–8.

165. Biant L, Bruce W, van der Wall H, et al. Infection or allergy in the painful metal-on-metal total hip arthroplasty? J Arthroplasty 2010;25(2):334, e11–6.

166. Molvik H, Hanna S, de Roeck N. Failed metal-on-metal total hip arthroplasty presenting as painful groin mass with associated weight loss and night sweats. Am J Orthop 2010;39(5):E46–9.

167. Perumal V, Alkire M, Swank M. Unusual presentation of cobalt hypersensitivity in a patient with a metal-on-metal bearing in total hip arthroplasty. Am J Orthop 2010;39(5):E39–41.

168. Watters T, Eward W, Hallows R, et al. Pseudotumor with superimposed periprosthetic infection following metal-on-metal total hip arthroplasty. J Bone Joint Surg Am 2010;92(7):1666–9.

169. Morlock M, Bishop N, Rüther W, et al. Biomechanical, morphological, and histological analysis of early failures in hip resurfacing arthroplasty. Proc Inst Mech Eng H 2006;220(2):333–44.

170. Witzleb W, Hanisch U, Ziegler J, et al. In vivo wear rate of the Birmingham hip resurfacing arthroplasty: a review of 10 retrieved components. J Arthroplasty 2009;24(6):951–6.

171. Griffin WL, Nanson CJ, Springer BD, et al. Reduced articular surface of one-piece cups: a cause of runaway wear and early failure. Clin Orthop Relat Res 2010;468(9):2328–32.

172. Barnes C, DeBoer D, Corpe R, et al. Wear performance of large-diameter differential-hardness hip bearings. J Arthroplasty 2008;23(6 Suppl 1): 56–60.

173. Fisher J, Hu X, Tipper J, et al. An in vitro study of the reduction in wear of metal-on-metal hip prostheses using surface-engineered femoral heads. Proc Inst Mech Eng H 2002;216(4):219–30.

174. Leslie I, Williams S, Brown C, et al. Surface engineering: a low wearing solution for metal-on-metal hip surface replacements. J Biomed Mater Res B Appl Biomater 2008;90(2):558–65.

175. Tharani R, Dorey FJ, Schmalzried TP. The risk of cancer following total hip or knee arthroplasty. J Bone Joint Surg Am 2001;83(5):774–80.

176. Tower S. Arthroprosthetic cobaltism: neurological and cardiac manifestations in two patients with metal-on-metal arthroplasty: a case report. J Bone Joint Surg Am 2010;92(17):2847–51.

177. Jacobs J. Commentary and perspective on: "arthroprosthetic cobaltism: neurological and cardiac manifestations in two patients with metal-on-metal arthroplasty. a case report". J Bone Joint Surg Am October 29, 2010 [online].

178. Daniel J, Pynsent PB, McMinn D. Metal-on-metal resurfacing of the hip in patients under the age of 55 years with osteoarthritis. J Bone Joint Surg Br 2004;86:177–88.

179. De Smet K. Belgium experience with metal-on-metal surface arthroplasty. Orthop Clin North Am 2005;36(2):203–13.

180. Stulberg B, Trier K, Naughton M, et al. Results and lessons learned from a United States hip resurfacing investigational device exemption trial. J Bone Joint Surg Am 2008;90(Suppl 3):21–6.

181. Vendittoli P, Lavigne M, Girard J, et al. A randomised study comparing resection of acetabular bone at resurfacing and total hip replacement. J Bone Joint Surg Br 2006;88(8):997–1002.

182. Amstutz H, Su E, Le Duff M. Surface arthroplasty in young patients with hip arthritis secondary to childhood disorders. Orthop Clin North Am 2005; 36(2):223–30.

183. Li J, Xu W, Xu L, et al. Hip resurfacing for the treatment of developmental dysplasia of the hip. Orthopedics 2008;31(12). Available at: http://www.orthosupersite.com/view.asp?rID=32924. Accessed December 20, 2010.

184. Phillips C, Barrett J, Losina E, et al. Incidence rates of dislocation, pulmonary embolism, and deep infection during the first six months after elective total hip replacement. J Bone Joint Surg Am 2003;85(1):20–6.

185. Beaulé P, Schmalzried T, Udomkiat P, et al. Jumbo femoral head for the treatment of recurrent dislocation following total hip replacement. J Bone Joint Surg Am 2002;84(2):256–63.

186. Smith T, Berend K, Lombardi AJ, et al. Metal-on-metal total hip arthroplasty with large heads may prevent early dislocation. Clin Orthop Relat Res 2005;441:137–42.

187. Kluess D, Zietz C, Lindner T, et al. Limited range of motion of hip resurfacing arthroplasty due to unfavorable ratio of prosthetic head size and femoral neck diameter. Acta Orthop 2008;79(6):748–54.

188. Malviya A, Lingard E, Malik A, et al. Hip flexion after Birmingham hip resurfacing: role of cup anteversion, anterior femoral head-neck offset, and head-neck ratio. J Arthroplasty 2010;25(3):387–91.

189. Williams D, Royle M, Norton M. Metal-on-metal hip resurfacing: the effect of cup position and component size on range of motion to impingement. J Arthroplasty 2009;24(1):144–51.

190. Bengs B, Sangiorgio S, Ebramzadeh E. Less range of motion with resurfacing arthroplasty than with total hip arthroplasty: in vitro examination of 8 designs. Acta Orthop 2008;79(6):755–62.

191. Ball S, Schmalzried T. Posterior femoroacetabular impingement (PFAI)–after hip resurfacing arthroplasty. Bull NYU Hosp Jt Dis 2009;67(2):173–6.

192. Gruen T, Le Duff M, Wisk L, et al. Prevalence and clinical relevance of radiographic impingement signs in metal-on-metal hybrid hip resurfacing. J Bone Joint Surg Am, in press.

193. dela Rosa M, Silva M, Heisel C, et al. Range of motion after total hip resurfacing. Orthopedics 2007;30(5):352–7.

194. Fowble V, dela Rosa M, Schmalzried T. A comparison of total hip resurfacing and total hip arthroplasty–patients and outcomes. Bull NYU Hosp Jt Dis 2009;67(2):108–12.

195. Le Duff M, Wisk L, Amstutz H. Range of motion after stemmed total hip arthroplasty and hip resurfacing. A clinical study. Bull NYU Hosp Jt Dis 2009; 67(2):177–81.

196. Lavigne M, Boddu Siva Rama K, Roy A, et al. Painful impingement of the hip joint after total hip resurfacing: a report of two cases. J Arthroplasty 2008; 23(7):1074–9.

197. Gerdesmeyer L, Gollwitzer H, Diehl P, et al. The minimally invasive anterolateral approach combined with hip onlay resurfacing. Oper Orthop Traumatol 2009;21(1):65–76.

198. McMinn D, Daniel J, Pynsent P, et al. Mini-incision resurfacing arthroplasty of hip through the posterior approach. Clin Orthop 2005;441:91–8.

199. Mont M, Ragland P, Marker D. Resurfacing hip arthroplasty: comparison of a minimally invasive versus standard approach. Clin Orthop 2005;441: 125–31.

200. Swank M, Alkire M. Minimally invasive hip resurfacing compared to minimally invasive total hip arthroplasty. Bull NYU Hosp Jt Dis 2009;67(2): 113–5.

201. Brooker A, Bowerman J, Robinson R, et al. Ectopic ossification following total hip replacement. Incidence and a method of classification. J Bone Joint Surg Am 1973;55(8):1629–32.

202. Back D, Smith J, Dalziel R, et al. Incidence of heterotopic ossification after hip resurfacing. ANZ J Surg 2007;77(8):642–7.

203. Rama K, Vendittoli P, Ganapathi M, et al. Heterotopic ossification after surface replacement arthroplasty and total hip arthroplasty: a randomized study. J Arthroplasty 2009;24(2):256–62.

204. Schara K, Herman S. Heterotopic bone formation in total hip arthroplasty: predisposing factors, classification and the significance for clinical outcome. Acta Chir Orthop Traumatol Cech 2001;68(2):105–8.

205. Fransen M, Neal B, Cameron I, et al. Determinants of heterotopic ossification after total hip replacement surgery. Hip Int 2009;19(1):41–6.

206. Vavken P, Castellani L, Sculco T. Prophylaxis of heterotopic ossification of the hip: systematic review and meta-analysis. Clin Orthop Relat Res 2009; 467(12):3283–9.

207. Neal B. Effects of heterotopic bone formation on outcome after hip arthroplasty. ANZ J Surg 2003; 73(6):422–6.

208. Neal B, Gray H, MacMahon S, et al. Incidence of heterotopic bone formation after major hip surgery. ANZ J Surg 2002;72(11):808–21.

209. Nayak K, Mulliken B, Rorabeck C, et al. Prevalence of heterotopic ossification in cemented versus noncemented total hip joint replacement in patients with osteoarthrosis: a randomized clinical trial. Can J Surg 1997;40(5):368–74.

210. Shields J, Mofidi A, Ward W, et al. Does a plastic drape reduce incidence of heterotopic ossification after hip resurfacing? Clin Orthop Relat Res 2010. [Epub ahead of print].

211. Back D, Dalziel R, Young D, et al. Early results of primary Birmingham hip resurfacings. An independent prospective study of the first 230 hips. J Bone Joint Surg Br 2005;87(3):324–9.

212. Clayton R, Beggs I, Salter D, et al. Inflammatory pseudotumor associated with femoral nerve palsy following metal-on-metal resurfacing of the hip. A case report. J Bone Joint Surg Am 2008;90(9): 1988–93.

213. Gay D, Desser D, Parks B, et al. Sciatic nerve injury in total hip resurfacing a biomechanical analysis. J Arthroplasty 2010;25(8):1295–300.

214. Patel R, Stygall J, Harrington J, et al. Intra-operative cerebral microembolisation during primary hybrid total hip arthroplasty compared with primary hip resurfacing. Acta Orthop Belg 2009;75(5):671–7.

215. Ball S, Pinsorsnak P, Amstutz H, et al. Extended travel after hip arthroplasty surgery. Is it safe? J Arthroplasty 2007;22(6 Suppl 2):29–32.

216. Yoo M, Cho Y, Ghanem E, et al. Deep vein thrombosis after total hip arthroplasty in Korean patients and D-dimer as a screening tool. Arch Orthop Trauma Surg 2009;129(7):887–94.

217. Daniel J, Pradhan A, Pradhan C, et al. Multimodal thromboprophylaxis following primary hip arthroplasty: the role of adjuvant intermittent pneumatic calf compression. J Bone Joint Surg Br 2008;90(5):562–9.

218. Nunley R, Della Valle C, Barrack R. Is patient selection important for hip resurfacing? Clin Orthop Relat Res 2008;467(1):56–65.

219. Witjes S, Smolders J, Beaulé P, et al. Learning from the learning curve in total hip resurfacing: a radiographic analysis. Arch Orthop Trauma Surg 2009; 129(10):1293–9.

Comparison of Fully Porous-Coated and Hybrid Hip Resurfacing: A Minimum 2-Year Follow-Up Study

Thomas P. Gross, MD, Fei Liu, PhD*

KEYWORDS

- Hip resurfacing • Hip arthroplasty • Metal-on-metal
- Uncemented • Cemented • Bearing surface

Surgeons have debated the relative value of cemented versus uncemented fixation in total hip arthroplasty (THA) for the last few decades. Because orthopedic surgeons have come to a general consensus on the superiority of uncemented fixation, uncemented fixation has virtually replaced cemented fixation in stemmed THAs in the United States.[1] Most acetabular components that are used today are of the uncemented type, as are about 80% of femoral stems. This trend is occurring in Canada and Europe as well.[1]

Hip resurfacing arthroplasty (HRA) has become an accepted alternative to stemmed THA in the last decade for young active patients wishing to return to a high level of activity, including impact sports. In modern metal-on-metal HRAs, hybrid fixation (uncemented acetabular and cemented femoral components) has been adopted as the standard.[2–4] Many studies have demonstrated successful early and midterm outcomes with survivorship rates of up to 97%.[5,6] In contemporary HRAs, cement technique has been shown to be quite variable and difficult to control.[2,7,8] Increasing cement thickness may cause more thermal necrosis and a higher risk of stress shielding.[8] Excess cement under the femoral component may result in leaving the femoral component incompletely seated; this extends the femoral neck, leaving uncovered reamed bone, and increases the risk of fracture. Also, the mechanical properties of the cement may result in an increasing rate of aseptic loosening over time.[9–11] Our results at the midterm (average 5.6 years) follow-up of the Corin (Corin, Cirencester, Gloucestershire, UK) Food and Drug Administration Investigational Device Exemption study of hybrid HRAs have demonstrated that cement fixation failure is the most common source of failure at a rate of 3%, accounting for half of all failures.[12]

Because of the superior results of bone ingrowth implants in stemmed THA, it may be logical to also apply uncemented fixation techniques to femoral resurfacing components. Several studies have reported positive clinical outcomes of contemporary metal-on-metal HRAs using nonporous uncemented fixation methods on both the femoral and the acetabular side.[13–15] We hypothesized that the clinical results of bone ingrowth type uncemented fixation on the femoral side in HRA should be equal to, if not superior to, cemented fixation at early follow-up. The purpose of this study was to report our 2-year clinical and radiological follow-up of the first modern fully porous-coated (uncemented) hip resurfacing prosthesis

No financial support is received for this study.
The author (T.P.G.) has received royalties from Biomet.
Midlands Orthopaedics, P.A., 1910 Blanding Street, Columbia, SC 29201, USA
* Corresponding author.
E-mail address: feilresearch@gmail.com

and to compare these results with those of hybrid hip resurfacing prostheses manufactured by the same company.

MATERIAL AND METHODS

The senior author (T.P.G) implanted the first fully porous-coated metal-on-metal Recap and Magnum combination hip resurfacing prosthesis (Biomet, Warsaw, IN, USA) in March 2007 (**Fig. 1**). The Biomet uncemented femoral hip resurfacing component has a full coating of titanium plasma spray under the entire undersurface of the femoral component, excluding the stem. The porous coating is identical to that present on the Magnum acetabular component and numerous other Biomet products. There are no other changes from the cemented version of the Recap device. The cemented Recap femoral component, used in the control group, has a grit blast cobalt chrome surface. The same instrumentation was used for both versions, which is designed to allow a 0.5-mm gap for cement and a press fit for the uncemented version. The Magnum acetabular component, used in both groups, has a full porous plasma spray titanium coating and 4 small radial splines. These implants and their instrumentation were described in detail in a previous publication.[15] Use of either the cemented or fully porous-coated Recap femoral component together with the Magnum acetabular component for an HRA procedure constitutes an off-label use in the United States; however, these implants are approved for total hip resurfacing in most other countries. Consent was obtained from each patient.

For the first year (from March 2007–February 2008), the manufacturer could not keep pace with the surgeon's demand for the fully porous-coated femoral implant. Implant type used in each individual case was therefore determined by the availability of the uncemented implant at the time of surgery. The decision regarding fixation type was made during the operation at the time of femoral preparation. If an uncemented femoral component of the correct size was available, it was used; otherwise, the cemented version was used. There was no supply limit of the cemented version. All the fully porous-coated and hybrid HRAs performed by the senior author during this period of time were included in this study. The surgical technique was the same for both groups, with exception of the fixation method on the femoral side.

All patients younger than 65 years who were otherwise candidates for THA and who had less than one-third of their femoral head bone stock missing and who had enough acetabular wall integrity to fix a screwless acetabular component were offered HRA (occasionally, older patients were accommodated if they insisted on HRA). It is not our practice to select patients for HRA based on implant size, gender, diagnosis, and presence of cysts or deformity.

There are no additional selection criteria for the type of femoral fixation (**Table 1**). No cases of uncemented femoral fixation were abandoned because of a failure to achieve adequate initial fixation or for any other reason. All cases had a tight initial press fit by manual testing, and none failed to seat at the desired level (within 1–2 mm of the trial position). In the cemented components, only

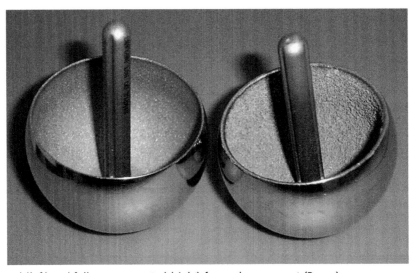

Fig. 1. Cemented (*left*) and fully porous-coated (*right*) femoral component (Recap).

Table 1
Summary of demographic and diagnosis data between fully porous-coated and hybrid HRAs

	Fully Porous-Coated	Hybrid	P Value
Surgical Date	March 2007–February 2008	March 2007–February 2008	—
Number of hips	191	96	—
Number of patients	182	90	—
Age at surgery (y)	50 ± 8 (range: 28–73)	52 ± 8 (range: 21–68)	.08
Weight (kg)	84.6 ± 16.2 (range: 49.50–132.75)	84.6 ± 18.0 (range: 51.3–167.5)	.93
Body mass index	27 ± 4 (range: 19–43)	28 ± 4 (range: 18–43)	.48
T score (Bone mineral density)	0.3 ± 1.6 (range: −2.2–5.2)	0 ± 1.19 (range: −2.1–2.8)	.10
Gender			.06
Women	50 (27%)	35 (39%)	—
Men	132 (73%)	55 (61%)	—
Side			.32
Left	92 (48%)	53 (55%)	—
Right	99 (52%)	43 (45%)	—
Diagnosis			.46
Osteoarthritis	133 (70%)	74 (77%)	—
Dysplasia	31 (16%)	14 (15%)	—
Posttrauma	8 (4%)	1 (1%)	—
Avascular Necrosis	12 (6%)	4 (4%)	—
Others	7 (4%)	3 (3%)	—

the undersurfaces of the component, but not the stems, were cemented. In both groups, cysts were treated in the same manner: grafting with platelet concentrate and acetabular reamings. No attempts were made to remove any femoral component (either type) after it was implanted. No patients scheduled for HRA were converted to THA intraoperatively for any reason.

By March 2010, all 191 cases in 182 patients who received the porous femoral component as well as the 96 cases in 90 patients implanted with the cemented femoral component reached their minimum 2-year follow-up. One patient (1 hip) in the control group died due to causes not related to his hip at the age of 57 years. Because we had his 2-year follow-up, this patient was still included in the study.

The posterior minimally invasive vascular sparing surgical approach using a 4-inch incision was used in both groups.[15] Platelet concentrate was used. A multimodal pain management program in combination with spinal anesthesia was used. A comprehensive blood management program was used that resulted in complete avoidance of any transfusion. Both groups were allowed weight bearing immediately after the surgery and advanced to impact sports after 6

months if desired. Patients were encouraged to proceed at their own pace using crutches for 1 to 2 weeks and then a cane for 1 to 2 weeks. They were encouraged to walk 1 mile daily without a support device by 6 weeks. No formal physical therapy was used after hospital discharge. Celebrex was used for 2 weeks postoperatively to avoid heterotopic ossification.

There were no statistical differences between the demographic characteristics in the 2 groups in terms of average age, weight, BMI, T score (bone mineral density), gender, side, and diagnosis (see **Table 1**). This confirms that similar comparison groups were created by this nonstandard method of patient selection.

Postoperative follow-up visits were requested at 6 weeks, 1 year, 2 years, and every other year thereafter and entered into our prospective database. Because 77% of the patients came from out of the state where the senior author practices, they were given 3 options to generate the clinical scores. They could answer the questionnaire related to their Harris Hip Score (HHS); visual analog scale (VAS) of pain score; pain location; and University of California, Los Angeles (UCLA) activity score during an office visit (32%), on an on-line database (55%), by mail (11%), or through a phone interview (2%). Radiographs were reviewed at each follow-up interval, but the latest radiographic review was used as a basis for this report. 76% of patients had complete follow-up information at a minimum of 2 years.

In this study, the null hypothesis for all comparisons between the 2 groups was that the evaluated parameter of the fully porous-coated group was the same as that of the hybrid group. The significance level α was set as 0.05. The statistical difference between numerical variables, including patient demographic information and clinical outcomes, was evaluated and compared between these 2 groups with the use of independent 2-sample student t tests. The statistical differences between categorical variables, including gender, operational side, and intraoperative complications, were also calculated and compared between these 2 groups based on χ^2 tests. The null hypothesis for all longitudinal comparisons within 1 group was that the evaluated preoperative parameter was the same as the postoperative outcomes. The comparisons between preoperative and postoperative HHSs in the same group were evaluated with the use of paired t tests. Kaplan-Meier curves were calculated to evaluate the survivorship rates of the 2 groups using revision of any component as the end point. The log-rank analysis was used to test the hypothesis that the survival functions between these 2 groups were the same. The data collection and analyses were performed with the use of OrthoTrack (Midlands Orthopaedics, p.a., Columbia, SC, USA) and JMP (SAS, Cary, NC, USA). The institutional review board approval was obtained for this study.

RESULTS

There was no difference in the survivorship rates between the 2 groups ($P = .92$). Specifically, there was no difference of the femoral complication rate. The femoral revision rate was 1% for femoral neck fracture and 1% for other early femoral failure in both groups. In both groups, Kaplan-Meier survivorships were the same: 97.8% using revision for any component as the endpoint, 97.8% using any failure of the femoral component as the endpoint, and 100% using any failure of the acetabular component as the endpoint at 3-year follow-up postoperatively (**Fig. 2**).

In the study group, 4 of the 191 hips (2%) required a revision of the femoral component. Two were revised because of femoral neck fractures (1%) at 1-month (59-year-old man) and 2-months (63-year-old man) follow-up and 2 because of femoral failure (osteonecrosis) (1%) at 10-months (50-year-old man) and 12-months (60-

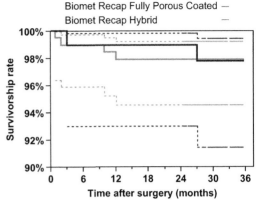

Fig. 2. Kaplan-Meier survivorship curves of fully porous-coated (uncemented) and hybrid hip resurfacing prostheses with 95% confidence interval. The solid lines represent the Kaplan-Meier survivorship curves. The dot plus solid lines represent the curve of 95% confident interval. Red indicates the group using Biomet Recap Fully Porous Coated HRA and blue, the group using Biomet Recap Hybrid HRA.

year-old) follow-up. In the control group, 2 of the 96 hips (2%) were revised: 1 was revised because of a femoral neck fracture (1%) (43-year-old woman) at 3 months postoperatively and 1 because of femoral failure (osteonecrosis) (1%) (31-year-old man) at 28 months postoperatively. All 6 revisions were isolated femoral revisions converting the resurfacing to a jumbo bearing metal-on-metal uncemented stemmed THA.

Other hip-related complications were seen in 2 of the 191 hips (1%) in the study group and 4 of the 96 hips (4%) in the control group ($P = .22$). In the study group, 1 hip dislocation (55-year-old man) was treated with closed reduction, but the hip was functioning well at the latest follow-up. One acetabular component appeared to be shifted in 1 hip before the 6-week follow-up (56-years-old man) postoperatively and remained stable at the latest follow-up of 2 years. The patient was functioning well at final follow-up. In the control group, 2 dislocated hips (both men, 44 and 46 years old) were treated with closed reductions. One deep infection with *Pseudomonas* (68-year-old woman) was cured with an open subcutaneous debridement and a 6-week course of intravenous antibiotics. The patient remains free of infection at the final follow-up of 2 years. One patient (68-year-old woman) suffered an abductor tear 4 months postoperatively that eventually healed after a platelet concentrate injection. All patients with complications were doing well at the latest follow-up visit.

There were no statistical differences in the average femoral component size, average blood loss, average hospital stay, and operation time between the study group and the control group (**Table 2**). The minimum duration of follow-up was 2.1 years for both groups (**Table 3**). In the control group, 1 patient had died (1 hip) due to causes unrelated to his hip surgery after 2 years of follow-up. At his 2-year follow-up, the patient's HHS was 97, UCLA score was 7/10, and VAS pain score on normal days and on worst days were both equal to 0. The clinical outcomes, including preoperative and postoperative HHSs and VAS scores, were summarized for both groups (see **Table 3**). The postoperative HHSs were significantly improved compared with their preoperative HHSs in both groups (P<.001).

Excluding the revised cases, radiological analysis revealed that no hip showed femoral radiolucencies or migrations in either group (**Fig. 3**). In the study group, there were 2 cases with reactive femoral lines without radiolucency adjacent to the femoral stem. There were 7 cases of focal femoral neck narrowing (superiorly at the head-neck junction) presumed to be caused by posterior-lateral impingement. There were 5 cases with Brooker I[16] and 1 case with Brooker III heterotopic bone. In the control group there was 1 case of Brooker I and 1 case of Brooker III heterotopic bone and 2 cases of partial 1 to 2 mm of radiolucency around the acetabular component.

DISCUSSION

Hybrid fixation with an uncemented acetabular component and a cemented femoral component has been the standard fixation technique in contemporary metal-on-metal hip resurfacing prostheses for more than a decade. This technique has achieved high success rates ranging from 94% to 98% at midterm follow-up, with the cemented femoral component achieving 97% to 100% success rates.[17–19] Using bone ingrowth rather than cemented fixation for femoral components is gaining popularity because of the long-term durability demonstrated for uncemented fixation in stemmed THA. Although metal-on-polyethylene hip resurfacing prostheses were abandoned largely because of a high failure rate as a result of wear debris, several studies reported successful bone ingrowth fixation of uncemented femoral components in these early hip resurfacing prostheses.[20–22] Two more recent studies have demonstrated promising results with uncemented fixation in early metal-on-metal hip resurfacing prostheses,[13,14] despite the fact that the femoral components were lacking a porous ingrowth surface. These results encouraged us to begin using a fully porous-coated femoral component in contemporary HRAs.

The purpose of this study was to evaluate the initial outcome of the first fully porous-coated metal-on-metal HRAs by comparing the clinical and radiological results of this implant at a minimum follow-up of 2 years with the results of a control group of hybrid HRAs performed during the same period by the same surgeon. Fully porous-coated femoral components for metal-on-metal HRA demonstrated a high success rate of 98% during the initial 2.4 years, equivalent to the early results using the same brand cemented femoral component. All the implants that did not fail because of femoral neck fracture or femoral head collapse showed stable radiographs without any impending signs of failure (radiolucency or migration) at 2 years.

We propose that femoral resurfacing prostheses that are radiographically stable at 2 years postoperatively should be presumed to be bone ingrown. In this study, the patients with uncemented components have clinical scores as good as those with cemented components at minimum 2 years. Survivorship reported in this study was comparable or better than the success rates that have been reported by other studies using hybrid hip resurfacing prostheses from other major HRA implant companies.[17–19,23]

We identified the following limitations of this study. Patient assignment was performed in

Table 2			
Summary of hospital data between fully porous-coated and hybrid HRAs			
	Fully Porous-Coated	**Hybrid**	**P Value**
Hospital Stay (d)	3 ± 1 (range: 2–7)	3 ± 1 (range: 2–5)	.9
Operation Time (min)	116 ± 21 (range: 80–220)	117 ± 15 (range: 90–169)	.9
Blood Loss (mL)	263 ± 100 (range: 75–550)	246 ± 96 (range: 50–550)	.18
Femoral Component Size (mm)	51 ± 4 (range: 40–60)	50 ± 3 (range: 44–56)	.22

Table 3
Comparison of latest follow-up outcomes between fully porous-coated and hybrid groups

	Fully Porous-Coated	Hybrid	P Value
Period of Follow-Up (y)	2.4 ± 0.2 (range: 2.1–3.0)	2.6 ± 0.3 (range: 2.1–3.0)	<.001[a]
Preoperative Information			
HHS	57 ± 13 (range: 22–83)	54 ± 13 (range: 21–81)	.07
Postoperative Information			
HHS	94 ± 9 (range: 55–100)	96 ± 6 (range: 70–100)	.25
UCLA Score	8 ± 2 (range: 2–10)	7 ± 2 (range: 3–10)	<.001[a]
VAS Regular Day	1 ± 1 (range: 0–7)	1 ± 1 (range: 0–7)	.48
VAS Worst Day	2 ± 2 (range: 0–10)	2 ± 2 (range: 0–9)	.89
Femoral Radiolucency	0 (0%)	0 (0%)	1
Incomplete Acetabular Radiolucency	2 (1%)	0 (0%)	.55
Number of Complications[b]	2 (1%)	4 (4%)	.22
Number of Failures	4 (2%)	2 (2%)	1
Deceased	0	1	.33

[a] P value is significant.
[b] Not including failed cases.

a nonstandard fashion. However, patients were not selected for femoral fixation type by the surgeon and all consecutive fully porous-coated and hybrid HRAs during this time period were included in this study. All other aspects of the surgical technique and perioperative management, other than the type of femoral fixation chosen, were identical for both groups operated on by a single surgeon during the same period. We therefore believe that the presented data provide an unbiased comparison between 2 types of femoral fixation that will be valuable to other surgeons.

The second limitation is that the results are preliminary and only show that the survivorship and complication rates of the fully porous-coated HRAs are equal to hybrid fixation at early 2-year follow-up. Most midterm clinical data on HRAs to date are based on hybrid fixation. It has not yet been demonstrated that the midterm and long-term follow-up outcomes of fully porous-coated technology on the femur will be better or worse than those of cemented femoral components for modern HRAs. Large clinical studies with longer-term follow-up using fully porous-coated femoral resurfacing components should be performed in the future.

Fixation of total hip implants to bone can be accomplished either by cemented or uncemented technology (bone ongrowth or ingrowth into a porous surface). Cemented fixation in THAs offers the advantage of immediate initial fixation

but the disadvantage of less-durable long-term fixation.[9,10] Cement fixation is achieved by an acrylic material (methylmethacrylate) that is brittle and that may induce an adverse biologic response.[11] Thermal,[24] chemical,[25,26] and possibly allergic[27] mechanisms have been shown to result in bone necrosis and subsequent formation of a fibrous membrane containing giant cells and histiocytes even in well-fixed implants. Cemented implants can gradually loosen from the bone over time because of an inflammatory reaction to particles caused by micromotion[28,29] and/or because of the gradual fatigue failure of this material.[30] This process may occur more rapidly in active patients and in implant situations in which the cement is stressed by shear forces rather than by compression forces.[31–33] Although cement technique has improved, a high degree of variability in the cement technique achieved in surgery still persists.[2,8,34] Cement fixation in stemmed THAs is increasingly reserved for older patients with more osteopenic bone, shorter life expectancies, and lower activity levels.[10,20]

In general, uncemented components achieve initial fixation to the bone by accurately preparing the bone so that the implant can be impacted with an interference fit. However, these components do require a period of 6 to 12 months of bone ingrowth before they are considered well fixed.[22] There is a small chance of bone ingrowth failure in uncemented implants.[14] However, if ingrowth occurs, it is durable and rarely fails in

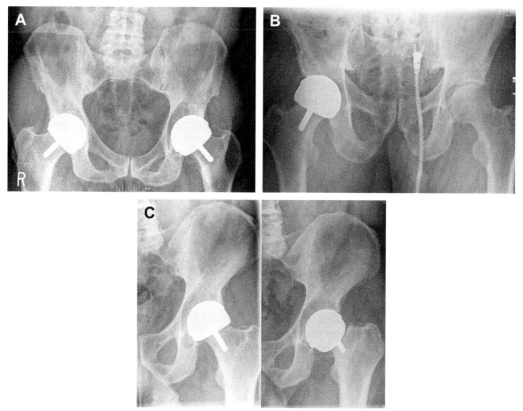

Fig. 3. (*A*) The 3-year follow-up radiograph in a 34-year-old man with primary diagnosis of osteoarthritis and HHS = 100 for both sides who underwent hybrid bilateral HRAs. (*B*) The 3-year follow-up radiograph in a 57-year-old man with primary diagnosis of osteoarthritis and HHS = 100 who underwent fully porous-coated HRA; focal neck narrowing is seen superiorly. (*C*) The radiograph in a 50-year-old man with primary diagnosis of dysplasia II who underwent fully porous-coated HRA with loosened femoral component at 10-months postoperatively (left, 6-week follow-up; right, 10-month follow-up). The femoral component has failed with varus collapse. Osteonecrosis is the suspected cause.

the long term.[14,35–38] One study of 2000 consecutive uncemented THAs between 1984 and 2001 found femoral stem survival to be 98.6% at 5 years and 10 years and 96.6% at 15 years with a mean follow-up of 5.5 years.[39] Other recent studies have demonstrated nearly 100% femoral stem survivorship with the use of uncemented fixation at 10 years.[35–38,40] Results of uncemented fixation in THAs have been reported to be superior to cement in young and active patients at midterm follow-up.[36,40]

In modern hybrid HRAs, cement has been demonstrated to be an excellent method for femoral component fixation at up to 11-years follow-up.[3,41] The best explanation that we can find for this phenomenon is that cement is loaded in a favorable fashion under a cemented femoral resurfacing component. On the acetabular side of all hip implants and around the stem in THAs, cement is often repetitively loaded with shear forces. Cement is known to perform poorly under

these types of loading conditions in the laboratory.[1,31–33] Under the resurfacing femoral component, however, cement is exposed to primarily compressive forces and is therefore exposed to ideal conditions to avoid fatigue failure. Although cement holds up reasonably well in femoral resurfacing component, we believe that it still may be one of the weakest links in the hip resurfacing construct and that it may be one of the primary causes of long-term failures in the future. Some surgeons have found cement fixation failure to be the most common failure mode in their studies.[12,42] Using uncemented fixation of both components in HRAs, therefore, seems to be a logical development.

In modern HRAs, there is a general consensus that uncemented fixation is superior for the acetabular component. However, uncemented femoral components have not been available until recently, and as a result, cemented fixation of the femoral component was used in most series of

HRAs. Katrana and colleagues[43] published a comparison of an uncemented Corin device with the hybrid Birmingham hip resurfacing and found no significant difference at 2 years. We previously reported no femoral failures in 19 patients at 7 years with this same implant.[14] Corin currently offers an improved uncemented femoral component, released in 2004 in England, with 3 longitudinal splines, partial titanium plasma spray coating, and full hydroxyapatite coating. We are not aware of any published data with this implant.

Cement fixation of the femoral resurfacing component is the current standard. Very little data exist to evaluate uncemented fixation of the femoral resurfacing component. To our knowledge, this is the first published report using a fully porous-coated metal-on-metal hip resurfacing implant. We have shown that there is no difference in the failure rates between cemented or fully porous-coated femoral components at short-term follow-up of 2 years. We believe that failure of any radiographic changes to develop after 2 years postoperatively demonstrates that bone ingrowth into the femoral resurfacing component can be reliably achieved. Learning from the principles of implant fixation that have been established over many years with stemmed THAs, we believe that uncemented fixation of femoral components in HRAs could be more durable after 10 years than cement, especially in the young and active patients typically selected for this procedure. Long-term analysis is necessary to validate this hypothesis.

SUMMARY

The purpose of this study was to compare clinical and radiological outcomes of the first 191 fully porous-coated HRAs with 96 hybrid HRAs performed during the same period at a minimum 2-year follow-up to evaluate the initial fixation of uncemented femoral resurfacing components. There were no differences in the failure rates between the 2 groups. There were also no statistical differences seen in the clinical scores of HRAs using either uncemented or cemented fixation on the femoral side. There was no radiolucency or migration observed in the fully porous-coated femoral components at minimal 2 years postoperatively. These results indicate that fully porous-coated femoral resurfacing components can routinely achieve reliable fixation and provide similar initial results as have been achieved with cemented fixation. Long-term results are needed to determine which type of fixation is superior for the femoral hip resurfacing component.

REFERENCES

1. Dunbar MJ. Cemented femoral fixation: the North Atlantic divide. Orthopedics 2009;32(9).
2. Mont MA, Schmalzried TP. Modern metal-on-metal hip resurfacing: important observations from the first ten years. J Bone Joint Surg Am 2008;90(Suppl 3): 3–11.
3. Amstutz HC, Le Duff MJ. Eleven years of experience with metal-on-metal hybrid hip resurfacing: a review of 1000 conserve plus. J Arthroplasty 2008;23(6 Suppl 1):36–43.
4. Schmalzried TP. Why total hip resurfacing. J Arthroplasty 2007;22(7 Suppl 3):57–60.
5. Daniel J, Pynsent PB, McMinn DJ. Metal-on-metal resurfacing of the hip in patients under the age of 55 years with osteoarthritis. J Bone Joint Surg Br 2004;86(2):177–84.
6. Hing CB, Back DL, Bailey M, et al. The results of primary Birmingham hip resurfacings at a mean of five years. An independent prospective review of the first 230 hips. J Bone Joint Surg Br 2007; 89(11):1431–8.
7. Campbell P, Takamura K, Lundergan W, et al. Cement technique changes improved hip resurfacing longevity—implant retrieval findings. Bull NYU Hosp Jt Dis 2009;67(2):146–53.
8. Ong KL, Manley MT, Kurtz SM. Have contemporary hip resurfacing designs reached maturity? A review. J Bone Joint Surg Am 2008;90(Suppl 3):81–8.
9. Stauffer RN. Ten-year follow-up study of total hip replacement. J Bone Joint Surg Am 1982;64(7): 983–90.
10. Chandler HP, Reineck FT, Wixson RL, et al. Total hip replacement in patients younger than thirty years old. A five-year follow-up study. J Bone Joint Surg Am 1981;63(9):1426–34.
11. Jones LC, Hungerford DS. Cement disease. Clin Orthop Relat Res 1987;225(225):192–206.
12. Gross TP, Liu F. Eight year clinic outcome of the metal-on-metal hybrid hip surface replacement. New Orleans (LA): AAOS; 2010.
13. Lilikakis AK, Vowler SL, Villar RN. Hydroxyapatite-coated femoral implant in metal-on-metal resurfacing hip arthroplasty: minimum of two years follow-up. Orthop Clin North Am 2005;36(2):215–22, ix.
14. Gross TP, Liu F. Metal-on-metal hip resurfacing with an uncemented femoral component. A seven-year follow-up study. J Bone Joint Surg Am 2008; 90(Suppl 3):32–7.
15. Gross TP, Liu F. Minimally invasive posterior approach for hip resurfacing arthroplasty. Tech Orthop 2010; 25(1):39–49.
16. Brooker AF, Bowerman JW, Robinson RA, et al. Ectopic ossification following total hip replacement. Incidence and a method of classification. J Bone Joint Surg Am 1973;55(8):1629–32.

17. Back DL, Dalziel R, Young D, et al. Early results of primary Birmingham hip resurfacings. An independent prospective study of the first 230 hips. J Bone Joint Surg Br 2005;87(3):324–9.

18. Amstutz HC, Beaule PE, Dorey FJ, et al. Metal-on-metal hybrid surface arthroplasty: two to six-year follow-up study. J Bone Joint Surg Am 2004;86(1):28–39.

19. Mont MA, Marker DR, Smith JM, et al. Resurfacing is comparable to total hip arthroplasty at short-term follow-up. Clin Orthop Relat Res 2009;467(1):66–71.

20. Shimmin A, Beaule PE, Campbell P. Metal-on-metal hip resurfacing arthroplasty. J Bone Joint Surg Am 2008;90(3):637–54.

21. Hedley AK, Clarke IC, Kozinn SC, et al. Porous ingrowth fixation of the femoral component in a canine surface replacement of the hip. Clin Orthop Relat Res 1982;163:300–11.

22. Amstutz HC, Kabo M, Hermens K, et al. Porous surface replacement of the hip with chamfer cylinder design. Clin Orthop Relat Res 1987;222:140–60.

23. Ramakrishnan R, Jaffe WL, Kennedy WR. Metal-on-metal hip resurfacing radiographic evaluation techniques. J Arthroplasty 2008;23(8):1099–104.

24. Sund G, Rosenquist J. Morphological changes in bone following intramedullary implantation of methyl methacrylate. Effects of medullary occlusion: a morphometrical study. Acta Orthop Scand 1983;54(2):148–56.

25. Galin MA, Chowchuvech E, Galin A. Tissue culture methods for testing the toxicity of ocular plastic materials. Am J Ophthalmol 1975;79(4):665–9.

26. Linder L. Tissue reaction to methyl methacrylate monomer. A comparative study in the rabbit's ear on the toxicity of methyl methacrylate monomer of varying composition. Acta Orthop Scand 1976;47(1):3–10.

27. Fries IB, Fisher AA, Salvati EA. Contact dermatitis in surgeons from methylmethacrylate bone cement. J Bone Joint Surg Am 1975;57(4):547–9.

28. Jasty MJ, Floyd WE 3rd, Schiller AL, et al. Localized osteolysis in stable, non-septic total hip replacement. J Bone Joint Surg Am 1986;68(6):912–9.

29. Willert HG, Ludwig J, Semlitsch M. Reaction of bone to methacrylate after hip arthroplasty: a long-term gross, light microscopic, and scanning electron microscopic study. J Bone Joint Surg Am 1974;56(7):1368–82.

30. Chwirut DJ. Long-term compressive creep deformation and damage in acrylic bone cements. J Biomed Mater Res 1984;18(1):25–37.

31. Aspenberg P, Herbertsson P. Periprosthetic bone resorption. Particles versus movement. J Bone Joint Surg Br 1996;78(4):641–6.

32. Mann KA, Bartel DL, Wright TM, et al. Mechanical characteristics of the stem-cement interface. J Orthop Res 1991;9(6):798–808.

33. Janssen D, Mann KA, Verdonschot N. Finite element simulation of cement-bone interface micromechanics: a comparison to experimental results. J Orthop Res 2009;27(10):1312–8.

34. Maloney WJ, Schmalzried T, Harris WH. Analysis of long-term cemented total hip arthroplasty retrievals. Clin Orthop Relat Res 2002;405:70–8.

35. Grubl A, Chiari C, Gruber M, et al. Cementless total hip arthroplasty with a tapered, rectangular titanium stem and a threaded cup: a minimum ten-year follow-up. J Bone Joint Surg Am 2002;84(3):425–31.

36. McLaughlin JR, Lee KR. Total hip arthroplasty with an uncemented tapered femoral component. J Bone Joint Surg Am 2008;90(6):1290–6.

37. McAuley JP, Szuszczewicz ES, Young A, et al. Total hip arthroplasty in patients 50 years and younger. Clin Orthop Relat Res 2004;418(418):119–25.

38. Epinette JA, Manley MT, D'Antonio JA, et al. A 10-year minimum follow-up of hydroxyapatite-coated threaded cups: clinical, radiographic and survivorship analyses with comparison to the literature. J Arthroplasty 2003;18(2):140–8.

39. Huo MH, Parvizi J, Bal BS, et al. What's new in total hip arthroplasty. J Bone Joint Surg Am 2008;90(9):2043–55.

40. Hooper GJ, Rothwell AG, Stringer M, et al. Revision following cemented and uncemented primary total hip replacement: a seven-year analysis from the New Zealand Joint Registry. J Bone Joint Surg Br 2009;91(4):451–8.

41. McMinn DJ, Daniel J, Ziaee H, et al. Results of the Birmingham Hip Resurfacing dysplasia component in severe acetabular insufficiency: a six- to 9.6-year follow-up. J Bone Joint Surg Br 2008;90(6):715–23.

42. De Haan R, Campbell PA, Su EP, et al. Revision of metal-on-metal resurfacing arthroplasty of the hip: the influence of malpositioning of the components. J Bone Joint Surg Br 2008;90(9):1158–63.

43. Katrana P, Crawford JR, Lilikakis A, et al. Femoral neck resorption after hip resurfacing arthroplasty—a comparison of cemented and uncemented prostheses. J Bone Joint Surg Br 2006;88(Supp II):234.

Failure Modes of 433 Metal-on-Metal Hip Implants: How, Why, and Wear

Edward Ebramzadeh, PhD[a],*, Patricia A. Campbell, PhD[a],
Karren M. Takamura, BA[c], Zhen Lu, PhD[a],
Sophia N. Sangiorgio, PhD[a], Jeremy J. Kalma, BA[a],
Koen A. De Smet, MD[b], Harlan C. Amstutz, MD[c]

KEYWORDS
- Implant retrieval • Hip resurfacing • Metal-on-metal
- Loosening • Wear • Failure • Revision

Modern metal on metal hip replacement bearings are often seen as a durable option for younger patients because they are stronger and considered to produce lower rates of wear and osteolysis.[1] The use of metal-on-metal bearings has increased since the introduction of large-diameter components for hip replacements and hip resurfacings, which offer protection against dislocation. Consequently, metal-on-metal bearings are reported to be second in popularity to polyethylene-on-metal bearings.[2] However, concerns remain regarding the potential biologic reactivity and long-term effects of cobalt-chromium alloy metal particles and ions, particularly in light of recent reports of soft tissue masses,[3,4] necrosis,[5,6] and systemic effects[7] of elevated ion levels. Although the incidence of these problems is thought to be relatively low,[8] there have been calls to severely limit the use of metal-on-metal bearings.[9,10]

Our research center has collected a large number of failed metal-on-metal implants, including first-generation McKee-Farrar total hip replacements (THRs), early generation hip resurfacings (McMinn; Corin Group, PLC, Cirencester, UK and Wagner;

Sulzer, Winterthur, Switzerland),[11] and a range of contemporary large-diameter modular THRs and hip resurfacings. In 2006, we published a retrieval study of implant failure modes in metal-on-metal surface arthroplasties and reported that aseptic loosening and femoral neck fracture comprised most failures.[12] We also reported that revision directly attributed to wear of the bearings was relatively rare.

The aim of this study was to investigate the modes of failure in a larger collection of metal-on-metal THRs and hip resurfacings and to examine the correlations between the reasons for revision and a range of patient and implant variables related to wear.

METHODS

Between 1991 and 2010, 433 metal-on-metal implant retrievals were collected at the Los Angeles Orthopaedic Hospital Implant Retrieval Laboratory from 35 surgeons. Of the 433 retrievals submitted, 9 were postmortem retrievals collected as part of an institutional review board–approved willed joint donation program.

[a] J. Vernon Luck Orthopaedic Research Center, Los Angeles Orthopaedic Hospital, University of California, Los Angeles, 2400 South Flower Street, Los Angeles, CA 90007, USA
[b] ANCA Medical Center, Ghent 9000, Belgium
[c] Joint Replacement Institute, St Vincent Medical Center, 2200 West Third Street Suite 400, Los Angeles, CA 90057, USA
* Corresponding author.
E-mail address: EEbramzadeh@laoh.ucla.edu

Orthop Clin N Am 42 (2011) 241–250
doi:10.1016/j.ocl.2011.01.001
0030-5898/11/$ – see front matter © 2011 Elsevier Inc. All rights reserved.

At revision, all components and periprosthetic tissues were fixed in 10% buffered formalin. The femoral resurfacing components were resected with a portion of the femoral neck, if possible. The components were then cleaned, photographed, and examined grossly.

Then, 185 femoral and 121 acetabular components were measured for wear depth using the Coordinate Measuring Machine (BRT 504, Mitutoyo, Aurora, IL, USA) using 300 to 400 points digitized over the surface of the implant. Wear was adjusted by time in vivo to calculate wear depth per year in micrometer per year for each component.

The following implant variables were analyzed: implant design or type and nominal ball diameter. The following patient variables were analyzed: patient age at implantation surgery, patient gender, time in vivo, and reason for revision. These variables were based on the revising surgeon's clinical assessment, which prompted the revision surgery, rather than the findings based on the retrieval analysis.

The presence of adverse local tissue reactions (ALTRs) was noted by the revising surgeon, which included osteolysis and/or fluid-filled or solid masses, whereas suspected metal hypersensitivity or allergy was determined after implant retrieval and histopathologic analysis.[13] If there was a fluid-filled or solid mass, the surgeon was asked to assess the size of the mass as small, medium, or large.

Representative pieces of periprosthetic tissue were embedded in paraffin blocks for routine sectioning and staining with hematoxylin and eosin. Each case was given a score for aseptic lymphocytic vasculitis-associated lesions (ALVAL) by one of the authors who specialize in orthopedic pathology (P.C.). The ALVAL scoring guidelines involved the assignment of points for the synovial lining integrity, inflammatory cell type and extent of tissue infiltration, and degree of tissue reorganization as a result of inflammation or necrosis, as previously described.[13] The presumptive diagnosis of metal hypersensitivity/allergy was assigned to cases that had a high ALVAL score (8, 9, or 10 out of 10) and when other causes for the unexplained pain, such as infection or excessive wear, were excluded.

In 97 cases, the radiographic variables analyzed included both cup abduction angle and cup anteversion angle measured from standard anteroposterior radiographs using the EBRA software (Einzel-Bild-Roentgen-Analysis, University of Innsbruck, Austria). In 157 cases, only the abduction angle was measured using standard anteroposterior radiographs, using the intertear drop mark to level the radiographs. Radiographs were not available for the remaining retrievals, and in some other cases, the radiographs either did not include the entire pelvis or did not allow for accurate measurement of the cup position angles.

Statistical analysis was performed using SPSS version 15 analytic software (SPSS, Inc, Chicago, IL, USA). Box plots were used to compare differences in continuous variables, followed by Wilcoxon rank sum tests to assess the associated statistical certainty.

RESULTS
Implant Types and Reasons for Revision

For the collection of retrievals in the present study (both THRs and conventional hip resurfacings), the most frequent reason for revision surgery was acetabular loosening (N = 102), followed by femoral loosening (N = 70) and femoral neck fracture of hip resurfacings (N = 63) (**Fig. 1, Table 1**). An example of a loosened acetabular component and a radiograph of a loosened femoral component are shown in **Figs. 2** and **3**.

Most of the retrievals were of Conserve® Plus (Wright Medical Technology, Arlington, TN, USA) metal-on-metal resurfacing implants (N = 111) because this site was contracted to evaluate all retrievals in the multicenter Food and Drug Administration trial. This retrieval was followed by the BIRMINGHAM HIP Resurfacing System (BHR, N = 81) (Smith & Nephew, Inc, Memphis, TN, USA). For these 2 implants, the most commonly observed reason for revision was femoral loosening. In contrast, for the McMinn first-generation hip resurfacing arthroplasty, the Metasul THR (Zimmer, Inc, Warsaw, IN, USA), the Wright Medical conventional THRs, and other conventional THRs, acetabular loosening was by

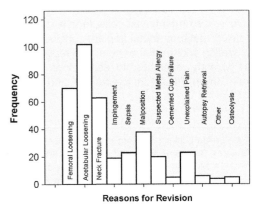

Fig. 1. The frequencies of various causes for revision surgery among the retrievals in the present study are shown.

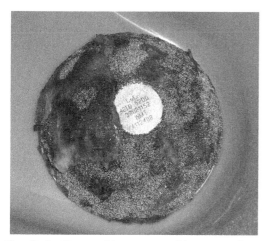

Fig. 2. A 42-year-old woman with osteoarthritis secondary to developmental dysplasia of hip received a 42-mm femoral/52-mm acetabular Conserve® Plus resurfacing system (Wright Medical Technology, Arlington, TN, USA). The acetabular component was positioned at 47.6° abduction and 17° anteversion. The acetabular component loosened and was revised 105 months postoperatively.

far the most frequently observed reason for revision (see **Table 1**). Among different types of resurfacing implants, the greatest number of femoral neck fractures was observed with the Conserve® Plus and the ASR (DePuy, Inc, Warsaw, IN, USA) retrievals.

Gender

Of the retrievals, 189 were from men and 201 from women. The gender was unknown in 43 deidentified retrievals. The reasons for revision were similarly distributed in both genders; acetabular loosening was the most commonly observed failure mode, followed by femoral loosening and femoral neck fracture. However, women had

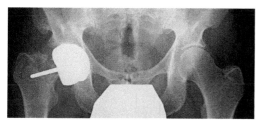

Fig. 3. Radiograph of the hip in a 51-year-old man with osteoarthritis who received a 52-mm femoral/62-mm acetabular Conserve® Plus resurfacing system (Wright Medical Technology, Arlington, TN, USA). The patient remained extremely active, playing hockey. The femoral component loosened after 139 months postoperation.

a higher frequency of acetabular loosening than men (60 vs 42) and a higher number of malpositioned cups that were abducted at more than 55° (30 vs 18) ($P = .19$). Women were more likely than men to be assigned a prerevision diagnosis of suspected metal hypersensitivity (20 vs 3) ($P = .0004$). Women had a significantly higher median cup anteversion than men (21.4° vs 13.6°, respectively; $P = .05$), but both genders had the same median cup abduction angle of 45°. There were 36 pseudotumors in 201 female retrievals, and 19 pseudotumors in 189 male retrievals. The incidence of pseudotumors was significantly higher in women ($P = .03$).

The median femoral wear rate per year was 5.25 µm/y in men compared with 6.3 µm/y in women ($P = .3$) (**Fig. 4**). Similarly, median cup wear rate per year was 4.37 µm/y in men compared with 5.71 µm/y in women ($P = .34$).

Design

It should be noted that wear was not measured in every component but, rather, was measured predominantly in those components for which high wear was suspected as a contributing cause of failure. Moreover, the distribution of wear was not normal because there were a few outliers for each type. For example, the mean femoral component wear per year in vivo was highest with the ASR, which was 19.7 µm/y, whereas the median femoral wear for the same ASR components was 8.6 µm/y (**Fig. 5**). The smallest mean femoral wear was found with the Metasul, 5.1 µm/y, and the median femoral wear rate with the Metasul was 4.5 µm/y. In contrast, the highest mean acetabular wear was with the BHR, 19.5 µm/y, comparable with that of conventional metal-on-metal THRs, 19.4 µm/y (see **Fig. 4**). The median wear values, however, were generally below 10 µm/y, whereas the BHR and the conventional THRs had median values of 9.9 µm/y and 10.2 µm/y, respectively. It must also be noted that the conventional THRs included some older-generation designs. In general, values of wear per year were higher for the cup than for the ball (**Fig. 6**).

Old Versus Current Designs

There were 67 early metal-on-metal resurfacing designs of McMinn, 2 of Wagner, and 167 of current-generation metal-on-metal resurfacing designs (Conserve® Plus, ASR, BHR, ReCap [Biomet, Warsaw, IN, USA], Cormet [Corin, Cirencester, England, UK], Durom [Zimmer, Warsaw, IN, USA]) in the collection. The median femoral wear rate was higher in the old design, which was

Table 1
Reasons for revision of M-M hip retrievals collected by the Orthopaedic Hospital Implant Retrieval Lab

	Femoral Loosening	Acetabular Loosening	Neck Fracture	Impingement	Sepsis	Malposition	Suspected Metal Allergy	Cup Cement	Unexplained Pain	Autopsy Retrieval	Other	Osteolysis	Total
BHR	21	8	8	3	4	20	10	0	7	0	0	0	81
Conserve® Plus	36	18	28	1	10	4	1	0	4	2	1	2	107
McMinn	6	18	3	0	2	0	0	5	0	1	0	0	35
Cormet	1	5	0	0	0	0	0	0	0	0	0	0	6
ASR	0	1	12	0	0	7	2	0	1	0	0	0	23
Durom	0	2	0	3	0	3	0	0	0	0	0	0	8
Metasul	2	19	0	5	2	1	3	0	4	2	1	0	39
WMT THR	2	16	0	3	1	0	1	0	0	0	1	0	24
Other Resurfacing	0	3	11	1	2	1	0	0	1	0	0	0	19
Other THR	2	12	1	3	2	2	3	0	6	1	1	3	36
Total	70	102	63	19	23	38	20	5	23	6	4	5	378

Abbreviation: WMT THR, Wright Medical Technology total hip replacement.

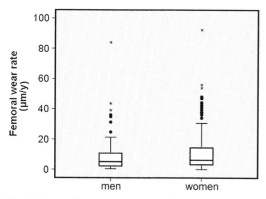

Fig. 4. Box plots representing femoral wear rate distributions in men and women.

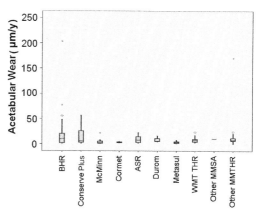

Fig. 6. Box plots representing acetabular wear rate distributions by design.

7.40 μm/y, than in the current design, which was 6.03 μm/y; however, this difference was not significant (*P* = .67). The median cup wear rate was higher in the current design than in the early design (5.37 μm/y vs 2.39 μm/y, respectively; *P* = .12).

Pseudotumors

The femoral ball wear was higher in failures with pseudotumors, with a median of 8.00 μm/y, than in retrievals without pseudotumors, with a median of 5.25 μm/y, (*P* = .057) (**Fig. 7**). The acetabular wear was also higher in retrievals with pseudotumors, with a median wear rate of 10.02 μm/y, than in failures without pseudotumors, with a median wear rate of 4.15 μm/y (*P* = .05) (**Fig. 8**). Cup abduction was significantly higher in retrievals with pseudotumors, with a median acetabular abduction angle of 52.0°, than in those without pseudotumors, with an angle of 44.1°

(*P*<.001) (**Fig. 9**). Median acetabular anteversion angle was also significantly higher in retrievals with pseudotumors (23.8°, pseudotumors; 18.9°, no pseudotumors; *P* = .052).

Cup Position Angles

Femoral component wear was higher in cases in which the cup was in more than 50° abduction, with a mean femoral wear rate of 21.7 ± 21.1 μm/y, than in cases in which the cup was in 30° to 50° abduction, which had a mean femoral wear rate of 5.7 ± 4.5 μm/y (*P*<.001) (**Fig. 10**). In addition, acetabular cup wear was higher in cases in which the cup was in more than 30° abduction, with a mean wear rate of 22.7 ± 41.0 μm/y, than in cases in which the cup was in 30° to 50° abduction, which had a mean cup wear rate of 9.8 ± 25.0 μm/y (*P*<.001) (**Fig. 11**).

Femoral component wear was very similar (although slightly higher) in cases in which the acetabular component was positioned at more

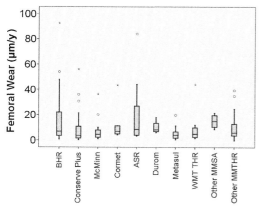

Fig. 5. Box plots representing femoral wear rate distributions by design. MMSA, metal-on-metal surface arthroplasty; MMTHR, metal-on-metal total hip replacement; WMT THR, Wright Medical Technology total hip replacement.

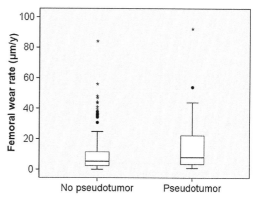

Fig. 7. Box plots representing femoral wear rate distributions for retrievals with and without pseudotumors.

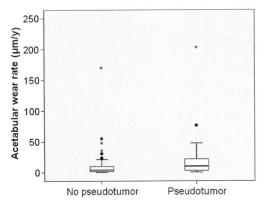

Fig. 8. Box plots representing acetabular wear rate distributions for retrievals with and without pseudotumors.

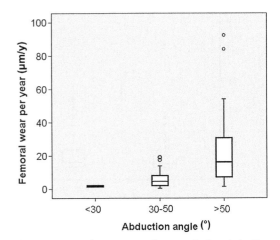

Fig. 10. Femoral wear rates by acetabular abduction zones.

than 25° anteversion, with a mean wear rate of 10.9 ± 12.6 µm/y, compared with cases in which the cup was in 5° to 25° anteversion, which had a mean wear rate of 9.5 ± 11.0 µm/y, and this difference was not significant ($P = .6$). Similarly, acetabular cup wear was higher in cases in which the acetabular component was in more than 25° anteversion, with a mean wear rate of 19.8 ± 20.8 µm/y, than in cases in which the cup was in 5° to 25° anteversion, which had a mean cup wear rate of 7.1 ± 11.0 µm/y, although the difference was not statistically significant ($P = .1$).

Suspected Metal Hypersensitivity/Allergy

In cases in which metal hypersensitivity/allergy was considered to be likely based on an ALVAL score of 8 to 10, the median femoral component wear rate was 3.42 µm/y, which was significantly less than in cases in which metal hypersensitivity/allergy was considered to be unlikely, median 6.9 µm/y

($P = .004$) (**Fig. 12**). The median acetabular wear rate was smaller in the group in which metal hypersensitivity/allergy was considered likely than in the group in which it was considered not likely (2.61 µm/y vs 5.38 µm/y, respectively; $P = .097$).

Patients with suspected metal hypersensitivity/allergy had a higher likelihood of having a pseudotumor (15 of 23 hips) than those without suspected metal hypersensitivity/allergy (28 of 330 hips) ($P = .0001$) (**Table 2**). However, among the cases with pseudotumor, more were considered to have failed for mechanical reasons than for metal hypersensitivity/allergy (see **Table 2**). Specifically, in 330 cases in which metal hypersensitivity/allergy was nearly ruled out, only 28 cases (<10%) were found with pseudotumors.

Among patients without suspected metal hypersensitivity, wear rates were substantially higher in

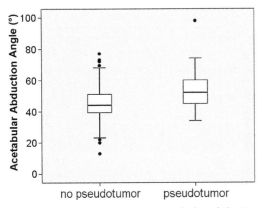

Fig. 9. Box plots representing acetabular abduction angle distributions for retrievals with and without pseudotumors.

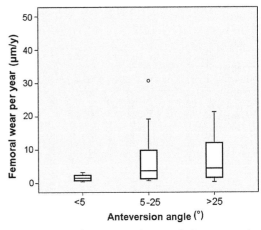

Fig. 11. Femoral wear rates by acetabular anteversion zones.

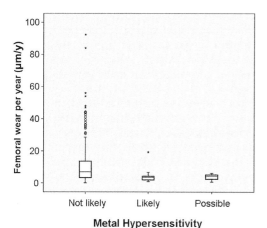

Fig. 12. Femoral wear rates for cases with and without suspected metal hypersensitivity. In some cases, metal hypersensitivity was not found to be probable but could not be ruled out; these cases were categorized as 'possible.'

Table 3
Femoral wear rate (μm/Y)

	No Pseudotumor	Pseudotumor Found
No Suspected Hypersensitivity	6	14.9
Suspected Hypersensitivity	3.40	3.42

press regarding their long-term benefits in light of some short-term failures.

A major limitation in our study was the variability inherent in using revision specimens for the analysis of covariate factors involved in the failure process and in the wear of the bearings. Although the surgeon coauthors (H.C.A, K.D.S) contributed nearly all the cases they revised for a wide variety of causes, many other specimens may have been submitted by others because the revising surgeon wanted to establish the cause of an unexplained failure. This reason would explain why we received a large number of cases revised for unexplained pain and suspected metal hypersensitivity. Joint replacement failure and bearing wear are both known to be multifactorial.[14–16] Although recognizing this fact, our analysis of a large number of specimens suggested that several of the many factors were likely to be more influential on both failure mode and implant wear than others.

Another limitation was in the assessment of wear using coordinate data from the scanned bearing surfaces. Specifically, we had no information about the preimplantation sphericity of the implants. Therefore, the initial surface of each implant was assumed a perfect sphere. However, the maximum initial allowable departure from a sphere for metal-on-metal hip implants is specified as 5 μm by ASTM F2033. In a hip wear simulator study of metal-on-metal specimens, Bowsher and colleagues[17] reported that the initial nonsphericity was from 5 to 10 μm in a group of Corin components. Older components may have even larger deviations from a sphere. Thus, the wear

those who had pseudotumors than in those who did not. Median femoral component wear rates are shown in **Table 3**, acetabular component wear rates, in **Table 4**. In contrast, among those with suspected metal hypersensitivity, wear rates were the same or lower in those who had pseudotumors.

DISCUSSION

The aim of this study was to investigate the modes of failure in a large collection of metal-on-metal THRs and hip resurfacings and to examine the correlations between the reasons for revision and patient and implant variables likely to be related to the amount of wear of the bearings. This study was performed at a time when metal-on-metal hip replacements were under increasing scrutiny in the orthopedic community and the popular

Table 2
Number of patients with or without metal hypersensitivity/allergy depending on the presence or absence of pseudotumor

	No Pseudotumor	Pseudotumor Found
No Suspected Hypersensitivity	302	28
Suspected Hypersensitivity	8	15
Cannot Establish	9	2

Table 4
Acetabular wear rate (μm/Y)

	No Pseudotumor	Pseudotumor Found
No Suspected Hypersensitivity	4.0	17.2
Suspected Hypersensitivity	8.4	1.3

depth estimation could potentially include the initial nonsphericity. This error would comprise a larger percentage for those implants with less wear. Another technical limitation was that although the wear in the areas near the edge was estimated, the wear on the acetabular rim per se was not measured because there was no accurate information on the initial rim geometry.

Retrieval studies have reported the cause of femoral failure from metal-on-metal resurfacings to be multifactorial; failure has been found to depend on factors such as varus positioning for femoral neck fractures,[18,19] component size,[20–22] implant positioning influencing wear and pseudotumor formation,[21,23] and implant design.[6] In previous studies of polyethylene-on-metal, Schmalzried and colleagues[14] demonstrated that polyethylene wear in vivo was multifactorial and found that patient and implant factors, operative technique, and fixation were related to polyethylene wear. Analogous relationships may exist in metal-on-metal implants.

Significant differences in femoral wear rates were found between the highest wearing femoral design (ASR) and lowest wearing femoral design (Metasul); however, the correlation for the cup wear rates was weak, most likely because fewer cases had cup wear measurements and because the ASRs in our collection were mostly revised for reasons other than acetabular malposition and so were less likely to have high wear. Implant design has been reported as an important factor in implant wear and failure because of differences in clearance and cup coverage angle.[6] Implant designs with smaller coverage angles place the implant at risk for edge loading, especially in components that are smaller in size and malpositioned.[24] Our group demonstrated in a previous study of a subset of the collection presented here, that malpositioned implants had a higher wear rate than well-positioned implants.[12] In other studies, significant positive correlations between both acetabular abduction and anteversion with metal ion levels[21,25] and with component wear[6,26] have been reported.

Our study found no significant correlation between femoral head size and component wear (both femoral and acetabular wear), although Langton and colleagues[21] found femoral head size to inversely correlate with increased ions, a reliable surrogate of wear.[25] McBryde and colleagues[22] found component size to be the best predictor for revision, with risk for revision increasing as head size decreased. Part of the reason for this apparent discrepancy may be the inclusion of many short-term failures, such as femoral neck fractures, in our group.

The patient factors analyzed in this study were age at surgery and gender. Although gender did not reach statistical significance, women trended toward higher femoral and acetabular wear rates. This finding has also been reported previously,[22] but because women generally have smaller implants, size rather than gender may be a stronger covariate.

This study was based on a varied collection of revised hip replacements submitted from a large number of surgeons. As such, there are further limitations to be considered. First, we cannot comment on the incidence of the failure modes that we describe because in most cases, we do not know the percentage of failures that the specimens represent within each patient cohort. Second, the reason for revision was not always consistent with the failure mode that was determined after analysis of the retrieved implant and tissues because these analyses provided information that was not available before surgery. However, the varied sources of our specimens likely represent the spectrum of clinical failures from surgeons with variable surgical skills and experience and therefore provide a suitable data set for the analysis of patient and implant factors. One exception is the group of retrievals from the surgeon coauthors (H.C.A, K.D.S) who have been able to closely follow-up their patients and therefore to calculate failure rates within the cohorts. For example H.C.A has reported an incidence of 0.6 of ALTRs in more than 1300 hips with a follow-up of 14 years, and K.D.S has reported 3 femoral neck fractures in more than 3000 hip resurfacing cases. Their reports are included in other articles within this issue.

Although there have been many concerning reports regarding the effects of high implant wear such as periprosthetic inflammation,[27] pseudotumors,[3] and osteolysis,[28] in our collection, the most prevalent reasons for revision were actually mechanical (which include femoral neck fracture, femoral and acetabular loosening, impingement, and acetabular malposition). This finding is supported by other studies in the literature. Morlock and colleagues[29] examined 267 hip resurfacing retrieval specimens, concluding that failures on the femoral side occur early (<9 months) and are associated with implant design and surgical technique. Most retrievals had been revised because of femoral fracture (66.5%) followed by acetabular loosening (9%), whereas revisions without cup loosening or fracture accounted for 25% of the specimens. In a registry data study of 5000 BHRs from 141 surgeons, Carrothers and colleagues[30] found femoral neck fracture to be the most common failure mode in the 182 hips that required revision, comprising 30% of the failures. In all, mechanical failures comprised most failures; acetabular loosening, femoral loosening, dislocation, acetabular malposition, and femoral neck fracture accounted for 65% of failures.

Using the Australian Registry data, based on 12,093 primary hip resurfacing surgeries performed between September 1999 and December 2008, Prosser and colleagues[31] used the Kaplan-Meier method and proportional hazards models to determine risk factors such as age, sex, femoral component size, primary diagnosis, and implant design in hip resurfacing failures. The investigators reported that components larger than 50 mm had a lower risk for failure than the smaller components, with men and women having similar risks of failure after adjusting for size. Some implant designs were found to have higher risk for failure than others. Femoral neck fracture and aseptic loosening/osteolysis accounted for 38% and 29% of all hip resurfacing arthroplasty failures, whereas metal sensitivity and unexplained pain accounted for 6% and 5% of the retrievals, respectively.

Our study supports the findings from the earlier-mentioned studies because the mechanical failures in our study accounted for most hip resurfacing arthroplasty and total hip arthroplasty revision specimens in our collection. This finding has not changed since our initial retrieval study in 2006[12] in which femoral neck fracture and loosening were the main causes of failure in 98 failed resurfacings. Our current study was expanded to include metal-on-metal THRs, and we still find that mechanical failures account for most failures. As other studies in the literature have reported, we also found wear and failure to be attributed to multiple patient and implant design factors, especially malposition.

One interesting finding in our study was a group of predominantly female patients with a variety of implant types that were revised for suspected metal hypersensitivity/allergy who were found to have, on average, low implant wear. Some of these cases also had pseudotumors, and the tissues were characterized by an intense lymphocyte-dominated inflammation that we have attributed to metal hypersensitivity/allergy. Proving metal allergy remains challenging in the absence of definitive clinical or histopathologic diagnostic criteria. It is unclear if all adverse tissue reactions are part of a spectrum of metal hypersensitivity/allergy or if a dose response exists. Kwon and colleagues[32] reported that lymphocyte reactivity to cobalt, chromium, and nickel did not significantly differ in patients with pseudotumors compared with those without pseudotumors, and they concluded that systemic hypersensitivity may not be the underlying cause of most pseudotumors. In the collection of retrievals and tissues we studied, there was only a weak relationship between wear rate and ALVAL score or pseudotumor formation. This finding indicates that further research is needed to clarify the relationships between implant and patient factors and the cause for failure of metal-on-metal implants, particularly those that may involve the immune system. Clearly, the failure process is multifactorial, and although high wear plays a role in many failures associated with component malposition, suboptimal design and mechanical processes remain the predominant causes for failure of metal-on-metal hip joint arthroplasty implants.

ACKNOWLEDGMENTS

This study was supported in part by the Los Angeles Orthopaedic Hospital Foundation, Los Angeles, CA, USA and by research grants from Wright Medical Technology, Arlington, TN, USA.

REFERENCES

1. Shimmin A, Beaule PE, Campbell P. Current concept review. Metal-on-metal hip resurfacing arthroplasty. J Bone Joint Surg Am 2008;90(3):637–54.
2. Bozic KJ, Kurtz S, Lau E, et al. The epidemiology of bearing surface usage in total hip arthroplasty in the United States. J Bone Joint Surg Am 2009;91(7):1614–20.
3. Pandit H, Glyn-Jones S, McLardy-Smith P, et al. Pseudotumours associated with metal-on-metal hip resurfacings. J Bone Joint Surg Br 2008;90(7):847–51.
4. Clayton RA, Beggs I, Salter DM, et al. Inflammatory pseudotumor associated with femoral nerve palsy following metal-on-metal resurfacing of the hip. A case report. J Bone Joint Surg Am 2008;90(9):1988–93.
5. Pandit H, Vlychou M, Whitwell D, et al. Necrotic granulomatous pseudotumours in bilateral resurfacing hip arthroplasties: evidence for a type IV immune response. Virchows Arch 2008;453(5):529–34.
6. Langton DJ, Jameson SS, Joyce TJ, et al. Early failure of metal-on-metal bearings in hip resurfacing and large-diameter total hip replacement: a consequence of excess wear. J Bone Joint Surg Br 2010;92(1):38–46.
7. Tower SS. Arthroprosthetic cobaltism: neurological and cardiac manifestations in two patients with metal-on-metal arthroplasty: a case report. J Bone Joint Surg Am 2010;92(17):2847–51.
8. Jacobs J. Commentary on an article by Stephen S. Tower, MD: "Arthroprosthetic cobaltism: neurological and cardiac manifestations in two patients with metal-on-metal arthroplasty. A case report". J Bone Joint Surg Am 2010;92(17):e35.
9. Lachiewicz PF. Metal-on-metal hip resurfacing: a skeptic's view. Clin Orthop Relat Res 2007;465:117–21.
10. Crawford R, Ranawat CS, Rothman RH. Metal on metal: is it worth the risk? J Arthroplasty 2010;25(1):1–2.

11. Amstutz HC, Grigoris P, Dorey FJ. Evolution and future of surface replacement of the hip. J Orthop Sci 1998;3(3):169–86.

12. Campbell P, Beaule P, Ebramzadeh E, et al. A study of implant failure in metal-on-metal surface arthroplasties. Clin Orthop Relat Res 2006;453:35–46.

13. Campbell P, Ebramzadeh E, Nelson S, et al. Histological features of pseudotumor-like tissues from metal-on-metal hips. Clin Orthop Relat Res 2010; 468(9):2321–7.

14. Schmalzried TP, Dorey FJ, McKellop H. The multifactorial nature of polyethylene wear in vivo. J Bone Joint Surg Am 1998;80(8):1234–42 [discussion: 42–3].

15. Callaghan JJ, Cuckler JM, Huddleston JI, et al. How have alternative bearings (such as metal-on-metal, highly cross-linked polyethylene, and ceramic-on-ceramic) affected the prevention and treatment of osteolysis? J Am Acad Orthop Surg 2008;16(Suppl 1):S33–8.

16. Shimmin AJ, Walter WL, Esposito C. The influence of the size of the component on the outcome of resurfacing arthroplasty of the hip: a review of the literature. J Bone Joint Surg Br 2010;92(4):469–76.

17. Bowsher JG, Clarke IC, Williams PA, et al. What is a "normal" wear pattern for metal-on-metal hip bearings? J Biomed Mater Res B Appl Biomater 2009; 91(1):297–308.

18. Shimmin AJ, Back D. Femoral neck fractures following Birmingham hip resurfacing: a national review of 50 cases. J Bone Joint Surg Br 2005; 87(4):463–4.

19. Vail TP, Glisson RR, Dominguez DE, et al. Position of hip resurfacing component affects strain and resistance to fracture in the femoral neck. J Bone Joint Surg Am 2008;90(9):1951–60.

20. Beaule PE, Dorey FJ, LeDuff M, et al. Risk factors affecting outcome of metal-on-metal surface arthroplasty of the hip. Clin Orthop Relat Res 2004;418:87–93.

21. Langton DJ, Jameson SS, Joyce TJ, et al. The effect of component size and orientation on the concentrations of metal ions after resurfacing arthroplasty of the hip. J Bone Joint Surg Br 2008; 90(9):1143–51.

22. McBryde CW, Theivendran K, Thomas AM, et al. The influence of head size and sex on the outcome of Birmingham hip resurfacing. J Bone Joint Surg Am 2010;92(1):105–12.

23. Grammatopoulos G, Pandit H, Glyn-Jones S, et al. Optimal acetabular orientation for hip resurfacing. J Bone Joint Surg Br 2010;92(8):1072–8.

24. De Haan R, Pattyn C, Gill HS, et al. Correlation between inclination of the acetabular component and metal ion levels in metal-on-metal hip resurfacing replacement. J Bone Joint Surg Br 2008; 90(10):1291–7.

25. De Smet K, De Haan R, Calistri A, et al. Metal ion measurement as a diagnostic tool to identify problems with metal-on-metal hip resurfacing. J Bone Joint Surg Am 2008;90(Suppl 4):202–8.

26. De Haan R, Campbell PA, Su EP, et al. Revision of metal-on-metal resurfacing arthroplasty of the hip: the influence of malposition of the components. J Bone Joint Surg Br 2008;90(9):1158–63.

27. Davies AP, Willert HG, Campbell PA, et al. An unusual lymphocytic perivascular infiltration in tissues around contemporary metal-on-metal joint replacements. J Bone Joint Surg Am 2005;87(1):18–27.

28. Carr A, DeSteiger R. Osteolysis in patients with a metal-on-metal hip arthroplasty. Aust N Z J Surg 2008;78(3):144–7.

29. Morlock M, Bishop N, Zustin J, et al. Modes of implant failure after hip resurfacing: morphological and wear analysis of 267 retrieval specimens. J Bone Joint Surg Am 2008;90(Suppl 3):89–95.

30. Carrothers AD, Gilbert RE, Jaiswal A, et al. Birmingham hip resurfacing: the prevalence of failure. J Bone Joint Surg Br 2010;92(10):1344–50.

31. Prosser GH, Yates PJ, Wood DJ, et al. Outcome of primary resurfacing hip replacement: evaluation of risk factors for early revision. Acta Orthop 2010; 81(1):66–71.

32. Kwon YM, Thomas P, Summer B, et al. Lymphocyte proliferation responses in patients with pseudotumors following metal-on-metal hip resurfacing arthroplasty. J Orthop Res 2009;15:15.

A Prospective Metal Ion Study of Large-Head Metal-on-Metal Bearing: A Matched-Pair Analysis of Hip Resurfacing Versus Total Hip Replacement

Paul E. Beaulé, MD, FRCSC*, Paul R. Kim, MD, FRCSC,
Amre Hamdi, MD, FRCSC, Anna Fazekas, MA

KEYWORDS

- Metal on metal • Ion levels • Differential hardness bearing
- Big femoral head • Total hip replacement

Recent improvements in metal-on-metal bearing technology have further led to the development of a total hip arthroplasty (THA) system that makes use of large-diameter femoral heads in both stem type and resurfacing hip arthroplasties.[1,2] Metal ion release remains a concern with using these bearings because of possible adverse tissue reactions and subsequent prosthetic loosening.[3,4] Recent reports have shown that metal ion release can be affected by bearing design, acetabular component orientation, as well as modularity due to fretting corrosion.[5–9] Although several clinical trials have shown relatively low metal ion levels after metal-on-metal hip resurfacing (HR) as well as 28-mm diameter Metasul (Zimmer, Warsaw, IN, USA)[10] and 36-mm metal-on-metal total hip replacements,[11] it is unclear if these studies can be applied to other implant designs as well as even larger-diameter metal-on-metal total hip replacements. Initial in vitro laboratory tribological wear testing have shown lower wear rates with the larger-diameter metal-on-metal bearings,[1,12] with further reduction in bearing wear being proposed using differential hardness bearings, which are intended to limit abrasive, adhesive, and surface fatigue damages.[13,14]

The primary purpose of the current study in this article is to measure metal ion release due to large-head metal-on-metal bearing by comparing HR with total hip replacement.

METHODS

The study was approved by and performed in accordance with the guidelines of the institutional review board. Informed consent was obtained from all patients included in this analysis. Twenty-six patients who received a modular stem type total hip replacement (Profemur® TL, Wright Medical Technology, Memphis, TN, USA) with a A-Class® differential hardness big femoral head (BFH) were matched on the basis of gender, femoral head size, and body mass index (BMI) with a group of patients who received the Conserve® Plus (Wright Medical Technology, Memphis, TN, USA) metal-on-metal HR implant (**Fig. 1**). The BFH and metal-on-metal HR groups did not differ on the matching variables: head size ($P = .083$), BMI ($P = .313$), or gender ($P = .337$). However, patients in the BFH group were older than those in the Conserve® Plus group ($P<.001$) (**Table 1**).

The Ottawa Hospital, University of Ottawa, 501 Smyth Road, CCW 1646, Box 502, Ottawa, ON, Canada K1H 8L6
* Corresponding author.
E-mail address: pbeaule@ottawahospital.on.ca

Orthop Clin N Am 42 (2011) 251–257
doi:10.1016/j.ocl.2011.01.005

orthopedic.theclinics.com

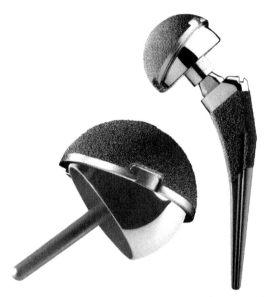

Fig. 1. Conserve® Plus HR and BFH A-Class® total hip replacement with Profemur® TL stem system. (*Courtesy of* Conserve® Plus; Wright Medical Technology, Memphis, TN, USA; with permission.)

The acetabular component was identical in both groups, which was a monoblock cobalt-chrome shell with a cobalt-chrome porous beaded surface. The acetabular components and the femoral components for the HR are made of a high-carbon cast alloy conforming to the ASTM F-75 standard. The castings undergo 2 heat treatment regimes before final machining and polishing. Hot isostatic pressing is done to eliminate tiny voids left in the castings during the cooling process. Solution annealing is done for the dissolution of large blocky carbides into the matrix. The A-Class® femoral head is made of a wrought alloy and has an open design with no modular sleeve and 3 different neck lengths. The stem used has a modular neck made of a titanium-vanadium alloy.

One 10-mm syringe of blood was collected from each individual at each assessment interval. Each syringe was labeled to indicate the sequence of collection. Before sample collection, all collection containers, syringes, and apparatus were triple acid-washed with Ultrex-grade chemicals and verified for absence of contamination by flushing with double deionized water, followed by analysis for residual trace metals. The samples of blood were maintained at room temperature until they had fully clotted (approximately 20 minutes) and then centrifuged at 1850g for 30 minutes. Serum and clot fractions were then separated, and the fractions were frozen and stored at −80°C in polypropylene tubes until analysis. All manipulations of the specimens were performed in a class 100 environment with a SterilGARD Hood (The Baker Company, Sanford, ME, USA) and class 100 gloves. All specimens were shipped to the Trace Elements Laboratory at the University of Western Ontario for elemental analysis using a high-resolution inductively coupled mass spectrophotometer.

The 2 groups were compared in terms of serum ion levels of cobalt and chromium at baseline and 6, 12, and 24 months postoperatively. The functional outcome at 2 years postoperation was assessed using the Harris hip score,[15] the Western Ontario and McMaster Universities Osteoarthritis index (WOMAC),[16] and the University of California, Los Angeles (UCLA) activity score.[17] Nonparametric Wilcoxon signed ranks tests were performed to determine differences in ion levels and functional outcome scores between the groups. Spearman correlation was used to measure the association between ion levels and BMI, age, femoral head diameter, and inclination, whereas Mann-Whitney U test was used to examine the relationship between gender and ion levels in both study groups (**Table 2**).

RESULTS

At the 2-year follow-up, the Harris hip score ($P = .03$) and the pain ($P = .049$) and stiffness ($P = .002$) subscale scores of the WOMAC were

Table 1
Means, medians, and standard deviations of demographic variables

Variables	A-Class® THR	HR	P Value
Gender (Men)	69.2%	80.8%	.337
	Mean, Median (SD)		
BMI	28.46, 28.00 (5.21)	27.24, 26.60 (3.81)	.313
Head Size	48.08, 48.00 (2.74)	48.31, 48.00 (2.51)	.083
Age	60.15, 59.00 (9.18)	54.38, 54.00 (5.96)	<.001

Abbreviation: THR, total hip replacement.

Table 2
Analysis of demographic variables and head size versus cobalt and chromium ion levels

| | HR (n = 26) | | | | Big-Head A-Class® (n = 26) | | | |
| | Chromium | | Cobalt | | Chromium | | Cobalt | |
Variables	r^a	P Value	r^a	P Value	r^a	P Value	r^a	P Value
BMI								
6 mo	−.21	.29	−.25	.23	.11	.64	.01	.99
12 mo	−.34	.11	−.34	.12	−.43	.08	−.13	.60
24 mo	**−.49**	**.01***	**−.45**	**.02***	−.12	.59	−.02	.94
Age								
6 mo	.17	.42	.12	.55	.16	.47	.41	.06
12 mo	−.09	.68	−.07	.75	.01	.99	.36	.14
24 mo	.07	.72	.11	.58	−.04	.87	.30	.18
Femoral Head Diameter								
6 mo	.03	.87	−.11	.59	.25	.25	.16	.48
12 mo	−.31	.15	−.30	.17	.06	.81	.40	.10
24 mo	−.25	.22	−.19	.35	−.03	.88	.16	.47
Inclination								
6 mo	−.17	.50	−.30	.23	.27	.42	.38	.26
12 mo	−.12	.65	−.31	.24	.63	.10	.03	.95
24 mo	−.01	.99	−.24	.35	.13	.69	.37	.24

| Mann-Whitney U (P Value) | | | | |
| | HR (n = 26) | | Big-Head A-Class® (n = 26) | |
Variable	Chromium	Cobalt	Chromium	Cobalt
Gender				
6 mo	.50	.20	.48	.42
12 mo	.37	.37	.56	.14
24 mo	.24	.31	.77	.42

Significant results in bold; * P<.05.
^{a} r, Spearman correlation.

higher for the HR group than for the BFH group. However, no significant differences were found in terms of the WOMAC function, the UCLA activity score, or the cup inclination (**Table 3**).

There were no significant differences in serum chromium ion levels between the groups at the 6-, 12-, and 24-month testing intervals; at 2 years, the median chromium ion levels were 2.40 μg/L and 2.58 μg/L for the HR and BFH groups, respectively (P = .615) (**Fig. 2**, **Table 4**). There was no association between serum chromium levels in either group and age, gender, head size, or cup inclination (see **Table 2**) Only BMI was negatively correlated with chromium ions at the 2-year follow-up in the resurfacing group ($r = -.49, P = .01$).

Cobalt ion levels were significantly higher in the BFH group at 6, 12, and 24 months (P = .002, P = .002, P<.001, respectively) than in the

resurfacing group. At 2 years, the median cobalt ion levels were 3.77 μg/L in the A-Class® THA group compared with 1.22 μg/L in the HR group (**Fig. 3**; see **Table 4**). There was no association between serum cobalt levels in either group and age, gender, head size, or cup inclination (see **Table 2**). As with chromium, BMI was negatively correlated with cobalt ions at 2 years in the resurfacing group ($r = -.45, P = .02$).

DISCUSSION

There has been an increasing use of metal-on-metal total hip implants in the last few years. Recent US data stated that 34.6% of all total hips implanted were metal on metal.[18] The reasons for this increasing use have been the ability to minimize the risk of dislocation with

Table 3
Means, medians, and standard deviations of outcome scores at 2 years

Outcome Measure	A-Class® THR; Mean, Median (SD)	HR; Mean, Median (SD)	P Value
Harris Hip Score	86.04, 92.95 (15.35)	95.26, 99.80 (7.92)	.030
WOMAC			
Pain Score	82.25, 87.50 (18.53)	95.00, 100.00 (9.24)	.049
Stiffness Score	66.88, 68.75 (21.94)	87.50, 87.50 (13.50)	.002
Function Score	81.54, 86.76 (18.28)	90.71, 97.06 (13.08)	.218
UCLA Score	6.83, 7.00 (2.23)	7.83, 8.00 (1.69)	.263
Cup Inclination	46.00, 45.00 (3.40)	46.94, 47.50 (4.28)	.108

Abbreviation: THR, total hip replacement.

the larger-diameter femoral heads[19,20] as well as maximization of the wear properties of metal-on-metal bearings.[1] Most early clinical series have been favorable,[21,22] however, certain implant designs had difficulties with initial acetabular component fixation.[23] In addition, the recent literature has shown that modular large-head metal-on-metal implants of certain designs were associated with higher metal ion levels as well as a higher incidence of adverse soft tissue reactions.[3] Although the authors found no significant adverse tissue reactions in their series, serum cobalt ion levels were significantly higher in the big-head metal-on-metal A-Class® THA group than in the HR group, whereas both the groups showed no difference in chromium metal ion levels.

In a randomized controlled trial, Garbuz and colleagues[5] compared large-head metal-on-metal total hip replacement with resurfacing arthroplasty and measured serum levels of cobalt and chromium in a subset of 30 patients, with both groups using the same bearing and acetabular component design. At 2 years, the serum cobalt level was 10-fold higher and the serum chromium level was 3.4-fold higher in the THA group than in the resurfacing group, with median values of 5.38 µg/L versus 0.54 µg/L for cobalt and 2.88 µg/L versus 0.84 µg/L for chromium. Similarly, Vendittoli and colleagues[6,7] also noted significantly higher cobalt ion concentrations at 12-month follow-up, with median whole blood values of 1.89 µg/L and 0.67 µg/L for BFH THA and HR groups, respectively. In these investigators' series, there were 2 types of femoral heads (closed with head diameter ≤48 mm vs open with head diameter ≥50 mm), and it was noted that the open design had a higher level of cobalt ion release of 67% at 12 months compared with the closed femoral head (whole blood median values of 3.06 µg/L vs 1.37 µg/L). In the authors' series, the serum cobalt levels were 4.4 and 3 times higher at 1 and 2 years in the A-Class® group than in the HR group, with values of 4.51 µg/L and 3.77 µg/L at 1 and 2 years in the A-Class® group and 1.02 µg/L and 1.22 µg/L at 1 and 2 years in the HR group. There were no significant differences in serum chromium levels between the 2 groups at any time interval. The cobalt levels decreased significantly at 2 years, which requires further follow-up to see if the trend remains. More importantly, no variable that was associated with higher cobalt levels except that of the use of the large-head metal-on-metal total hip bearing (see **Table 2**) was found.

The use of metal-on-metal bearings certainly brings into light the contribution of passive corrosion to the release of metal ions.[24,25] Although most orthopedic implants undergo some sort of surface treatment, such as passivation, corrosion

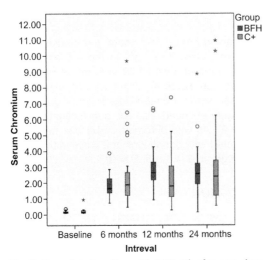

Fig. 2. Box plots (median with 95% CI) of serum chromium ion levels in BFH and Conserve® Plus (C+) groups at baseline and 6, 12, and 24 months.

Table 4
Means and medians of serum chromium and cobalt ion levels at each testing interval

Interval	A-Class® THR; Mean, Median (Minimum, Maximum)	HR; Mean, Median (Minimum, Maximum)	P Value
Chromium			
Baseline	0.18, 0.16 (0.10, 0.36)	0.21, 0.16 (0.10, 0.93)	.968
6 mo	1.79, 1.64 (0.73, 3.87)	2.55, 1.88 (0.46, 9.67)	.390
12 mo	2.95, 2.63 (0.92, 6.69)	2.52, 1.79 (0.28, 10.49)	.215
24 mo	2.83, 2.58 (0.14, 8.86)	3.05, 2.41 (0.55, 10.95)	.615
Cobalt			
Baseline	0.12, 0.09 (0.05, 0.57)	0.09, 0.08 (0.04, 0.19)	.469
6 mo	3.52, 3.26 (0.48, 10.25)	1.43, 1.12 (0.40, 5.09)	.002
12 mo	5.12, 4.51 (0.76, 12.85)	1.73, 1.02 (0.31, 7.42)	.002
24 mo	4.02, 3.77 (0.23, 9.59)	1.99, 1.22 (0.44. 7.13)	<.001

Abbreviation: THR, total hip replacement.

can still occur when the oxide layer covering the implant is ruptured from the metal substrate and unoxidized metal is exposed to physiologic solution, which permits an exchange of metal ions and electrodes, that is, corrosion.[24] The released metal ions can then form organometallic complexes that can activate an inflammatory response leading to osteolysis.[25] The extent and duration of the oxidation before repassivation varies based on the metal substrate and the physiologic environment. The observation of higher ion levels with the open femoral head designs in the study by Vendittoli and colleagues[6] and in the authors' series in patients who underwent A-Class® total hip replacement that uses the same design supports the concept of the greater surface area

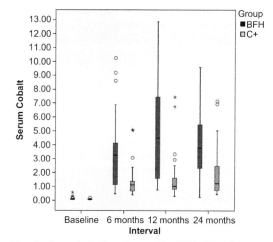

Fig. 3. Box plots (median with 95% CI) of serum cobalt ion levels in BFH and Conserve® Plus (C+) groups at baseline and 6, 12, and 24 months.

being exposed to the synovial fluid leading to a more significant corrosive process. This concept is also supported by the lower ion levels reported by Vendittoli and colleagues[10] using the 28-mm Metasul bearing. There was no significant difference in chromium levels in both the studies by Vendittoli and colleagues and by the authors'. A limitation of both of these studies is that neither was randomized, which may have had an influence on the clinical functional scores, with the patients who underwent hip resurfacing doing significantly better on the Harris hip score in the authors' clinical series. This limitation is, however, unlikely to have been a factor in the significantly different cobalt ion levels between the 2 groups.

Although hip simulator wear studies have shown a decrease in the wear rate with the use of the A-Class® differential hardness bearing,[13] the authors' results suggest that this may not translate into lower serum cobalt ion levels. These findings as well as that by Garbuz and colleagues[5] and Vendittoli and colleagues[6] emphasize the multiple possible sources of metallic debris with modularity[26] and implant design playing critical roles. More importantly, regarding the use of large-diameter femoral heads with metal-metal bearings, it seems that HR may represent the safest type of implant design in regard to metal ion release, which would also translate into lesser risk of an adverse soft tissue reaction.[3] The authors' data cannot be used to differentiate the wear performance of this differential hardness bearing because the source of the metal ions is not limited to the bearing. Consequently, a clinical series looking at this differential hardness bearing with an HR implant provides a clearer clinical picture of the potential benefits of this bearing. Continued close clinical follow-up of this series is required and the use of large-head metal-on-metal bearings should probably be limited to HR designs until the effect of the corrosive process with total hip replacements using large heads is better understood.

SUMMARY

This metal ion study comparing HR to large head metal-on-metal total hip replacement has shown significantly higher levels of cobalt at 1 and 2 years in the large total hip group but which were decreasing at 2 years. No difference was noted for chromium levels between the resurfacing and large head metal-on-metal groups. More importantly, this clinical data on higher serum ions with large head metal-on-metal total hip replacements is supported by 2 other clinical series. The use of a differential hardness bearing with a large head metal-on-metal total hip replacement does not seem to offer any advantage in regard to metal ion release; however, no conclusions for it in HR because of the confounding variable of passive corrosion in this open design BFH. Further clinical follow-up is required to determine the clinical significance of these elevated levels of cobalt ions in serum.

ACKNOWLEDGMENTS

The authors gratefully acknowledge the assistance of Heather Bélanger, RN, BScN and Gillian Parker, BSc (Ottawa Hospital, General Campus, Ottawa, ON, Canada) for their assistance with data collection and the coordination of this research project.

REFERENCES

1. Rieker CB, Schon R, Liebentritt G, et al. Influence of the clearance on in-vitro tribology of large diameter metal-on-metal articulations pertaining to resurfacing hip implants. Orthop Clin North Am 2005;36(2): 135–42.
2. Beaule PE, Mussett SA, Medley JB. Metal-on-metal bearings in total hip arthroplasty. Instr Course Lect 2010;59:17–25.
3. Langton DJ, Jameson SS, Joyce TJ, et al. Early failure of metal-on-metal bearings in hip resurfacing and large-diameter total hip replacement. A consequence of excess wear. J Bone Joint Surg Br 2010;92:38–46.
4. Campbell PA, Shen F-W, McKellop HA. Biologic and tribologic considerations of alternative bearing surfaces. Clin Orthop 2004;418:98–111.
5. Garbuz DS, Tanzer M, Greidanus NV, et al. The John Charnley Award: metal-on-metal hip resurfacing versus large-diameter head metal-on-metal total hip arthroplasty: a randomized clinical trial. Clin Orthop Relat Res 2010;468:318–25.
6. Vendittoli PA, Amzica T, Roy AG, et al. Metal ion release with large-diameter metal-on-metal hip arthroplasty. J Arthroplasty 2011;26(2):282–8.
7. Vendittoli PA, Mottard S, Roy AG, et al. Chromium and cobalt ion release following the Durom high carbon content, forged metal-on-metal surface replacement of the hip. J Bone Joint Surg Br 2007; 89:441–8.
8. De Haan R, Pattyn C, Gill HS, et al. Correlation between inclination of the acetabular component and metal ion levels in metal-on-metal hip resurfacing replacement. J Bone Joint Surg Br 2008;90: 1291–7.
9. Isaac GH, Thompson J, Williams S, et al. Metal-on-metal bearing surfaces: materials, manufacture, design optimization and alternatives. Proc Inst Mech Eng H 2006;220:119–33.
10. Vendittoli PA, Roy A, Mottard S, et al. Metal ion release from bearing wear and corrosion with 28 mm and large-diameter metal-on-metal bearing articulations: a follow-up study. J Bone Joint Surg Br 2010;92:12–9.
11. Engh CA Jr, MacDonald SJ, Sritulanondha S, et al. 2008 John Charnley Award: metal ion levels after metal-on-metal total hip arthroplasty: a randomized trial. Clin Orthop Relat Res 2009;467:101–11.
12. Dowson D, Hardaker C, Flett M, et al. A hip joint simulator study of the performance of metal-on-metal joints. Part II: design. J Arthroplasty 2004; 19(8 Suppl 3):124–30.
13. Barnes CL, Nambu S, Carroll M, et al. Differential hardness bearings in hip arthroplasty. J Surg Orthop Adv 2008;17:40–4.
14. Firkins PJ, Tipper JL, Ingham E, et al. A novel low wearing differential hardness, ceramic-on-metal hip joint prosthesis. J Biomech 2001;34:1291–8.
15. Harris WH. Traumatic arthritis of the hip after dislocation and acetabular fractures: treatment by mold arthroplasty. An end result study using a new method of result evaluation. J Bone Joint Surg Am 1969;51: 737–55.
16. Bellamy N, Buchanan WW, Goldsmith CH. Validation study of WOMAC: a health status instrument for measuring clinically important patient relevant outcomes following total or knee arthroplasty in osteoarthritis. J Orthop Rheumatol 1988;1:95–108.
17. Beaule PE, Dorey FJ, Le Duff MJ, et al. The value of patient activity level in clinical outcome of total hip arthroplasty. J Arthroplasty 2006;21:547–52.
18. Bozic KJ, Kurtz S, Lau E, et al. The epidemiology of bearing surface usage in total hip arthroplasty in the United States. J Bone Joint Surg Am 2009;91:1614–20.

19. Amstutz HC, LeDuff M, Beaule PE. Prevention and treatment of dislocation after total hip replacement using large diameter balls. Clin Orthop Relat Res 2004;429:108–16.

20. Cuckler JM, Moore KD, Lombardi AVJ, et al. Large versus small femoral heads in metal-on-metal total hip arthroplasty. J Arthroplasty 2004;19(8 Suppl 3):41–4.

21. Peters CL, McPherson EJ, Jackson JD, et al. Reduction in early dislocation rate with large-diameter femoral heads in primary total hip arthroplasty. J Arthroplasty 2007;22:140–4.

22. Engh CA Jr, Ho H, Engh CA. Metal-on-metal hip arthroplasty: does early clinical outcome justify the chance of an adverse local tissue reaction? Clin Orthop Relat Res 2010;468:406–12.

23. Berton C, Girard J, Krantz N, et al. The Durom large diameter head acetabular component: early results with a large-diameter metal-on-metal bearing. J Bone Joint Surg Br 2010;92:202–8.

24. Jacobs JJ, Gilbert JL, Urban RM. Corrosion of metal orthopaedic implants. Current concepts review. J Bone Joint Surg Am 1998;80:268–82.

25. Cadosch D, Chan E, Gautschi OP, et al. Metal is not inert: role of metal ions released by biocorrosion in aseptic loosening—current concepts. J Biomed Mater Res 2009;91:1252–62.

26. Bobyn JD, Tanzer M, Krygier JJ, et al. Concerns with modularity in total hip arthroplasty. Clin Orthop Relat Res 1994;298:27–36.

Revisions of Metal-on-Metal Hip Resurfacing: Lessons Learned and Improved Outcome

Koen A. De Smet, MD[a],*,
Catherine Van Der Straeten, MD[b],
Maarten Van Orsouw, MD[a], Rachid Doubi, MD[a],
Katrien Backers, PhD[a], George Grammatopoulos, MD[c]

KEYWORDS

- Revision hip arthroplasty • Hip resurfacing
- Metal ions • Outcome

In the last 15 years, metal-on-metal hip resurfacing arthroplasty (MoMHRA) has been used in increasing numbers to treat hip pathologies especially in young and active patients, with an estimated 500,000 third-generation MoMHRA performed to date. Arthroplasty registries have reported inferior survivorship of certain hip resurfacing designs,[1,2] recently leading to the withdrawal of the Articular Surface Replacement (ASR) design (DePuy, Warsaw, IN) from the market. Besides these reports, increasing numbers of revisions for unexplained pain and soft tissue reactions have been published,[3,4] potentially alerting the attitudes of the orthopedic community, health authorities, and the public toward MoMHRA. Although global consensus exists regarding the importance of implant design[5,6] and indications[7,8] for MoMHRA, the methods to follow-up MoMHRA patients differ.[9] More specifically, the measurement of metal ions in the peripheral blood has been recognized as a valuable and necessary tool to recognize increased wear of the articulating surfaces at an early stage,[9–11] and can be used as a screening method.

Ease of revision with minimal bone loss has been put forward as a theoretical advantage of hip resurfacing. Isolated failure of the femoral resurfacing component was safely and successfully converted to total hip arthroplasty (THA) in one series.[12] Another series highlighted the difference in outcome with different indications for revision.[4] Cases revised for fracture, avascular necrosis (AVN), or component loosening, that is, mechanical failures without soft tissue damage, had better outcome and lower complication rates compared with cases with pseudotumor and extensive soft tissue destruction.[4]

A review of 397 revisions of MoMHRA from the Australian Joint Replacement Register (AJR),[12] comparing survival as a mode of outcome for different types of MoMHRA revisions, confirmed that the best outcome was achieved with either femoral-only revision or revision of both components. However, even femoral-only revisions had twice the risk of revision of a primary THA. Acetabular-only revisions were reported to have a high risk of re-revision in the AJR, with a 5-year cumulative revision rate of 20%.[12]

The authors have nothing to disclose.

[a] Department of Orthopedic Surgery, ANCA Medical Center, Krijgslaan 181, 9000 Ghent, Belgium
[b] Independent Consultant Clinical Research, Bosstraat 19, 9830 Sint-Martens-Latem, Ghent, Belgium
[c] Nuffield Department of Orthopaedics, Rheumatology and Musculoskeletal Sciences, Botnar Research Centre, University of Oxford, Windmill Road, Oxford, OX3 7LD, UK
* Corresponding author.
E-mail address: dr.desmet@heup.be

Orthop Clin N Am 42 (2011) 259–269
doi:10.1016/j.ocl.2011.01.003
0030-5898/11/$ – see front matter © 2011 Elsevier Inc. All rights reserved.

The aim of this retrospective, consecutive case series of a single surgeon was to assess the outcome following revision of MoMHRA. In addition, the authors assessed whether the lessons learned from the initial previously reported experience[13] improved outcome, and whether screening with the use of metal ions had an effect on post-revision outcome.

PATIENTS AND METHODS

Between November 2000 and September 2010, the senior surgeon (K.A.DeS.) performed 113 consecutive revisions of failed metal-on-metal hip resurfacing arthroplasties in 110 patients. There were 3 bilateral revisions and 2 re-revisions of hip resurfacings where initially only the acetabular component had been revised. Of the primary 113 hip resurfacing procedures, 70 had been performed elsewhere and 43 by the senior surgeon (K.A.DeS.). The initial operations were performed between June 1996 and December 2009.

The number of revisions of hip resurfacings is increasing as more HRA are being implanted worldwide. In the authors' center, the number of revisions has risen from an average of 2 cases per year during the period of 2000 to 2004 to an average of 17 per year in the period 2005 to 2009 (**Fig. 1**).

Patient Demographics

There were 44 male patients (40%) undergoing 45 revisions (1 re-revision) and 66 female patients (60%) undergoing 70 revisions (3 bilateral revisions and 1 re-revision) (**Table 1**). The mean age of the patients at the primary hip resurfacing operation was 49.9 years (range 14–71 years) and their

mean age at the revision was 52.5 years (range 18–71 years). Forty-three of the primary MoMHRA were performed at the authors' center (38%). A total of 3313 MoMHRAs have been performed since 1998, resulting in a known revision rate of 1.5% (patients revised at this center and reported from elsewhere). The remaining 70 failed MoMHRAs (62%) were from elsewhere, with patients having had their primary surgeries in 50 different centers in 6 different countries.

The original diagnosis was osteoarthritis in 97 cases (85.8%), congenital hip dysplasia in 7 females (6.2%), avascular necrosis in 8 cases (7.1%) including 4 males and 4 females, and rheumatoid arthritis in 1 male patient (0.9%).

Revised Hip Resurfacing Types

The consecutive series of 113 revised hip resurfacing arthroplasties consisted of 63 Birmingham Hip Resurfacings (BHR) (Smith & Nephew, Memphis, TN, USA), 2 McMinn (Corin, Cirencester, UK), 19 Conserve® Plus (Wright Medical Technology, Arlington, TN, USA), 1 Conserve® Plus A-Class® (Wright Medical Technology), 10 ASR (DePuy, Warsaw, IN, USA), 10 DUROM (Zimmer, Winterthur, Switzerland), 4 ADEPT (Finsbury Orthopaedics, Leatherhead, UK), 3 CORMET 2000 (Corin), and 3 RECAP (Biomet, Warsaw, IN, USA) hip resurfacing arthroplasties (see **Table 1**). Two BHR had to be re-revised. Primary hip resurfacing procedures by the senior surgeon (K.A.DeS.) included 31 BHR, 8 Conserve® Plus, 1 Conserve® Plus A-Class®, 2 ASR, and 1 RECAP (see **Table 1**). The mean interval between the primary hip resurfacing operation and the first revision was 30.9 months (range 0–101

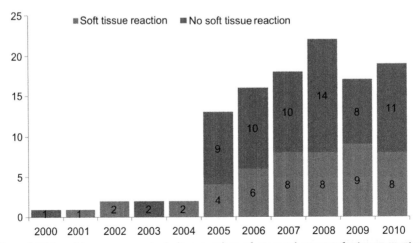

Fig. 1. Number of HRA revisions per year including number of cases where a soft tissue reaction was found intraoperatively.

Table 1
Demographics of patients and revised hip resurfacing implants

Number of revisions: N = 113	Bilateral revisions: n = 3 Re-revisions: n = 2	—

Patients: N = 110
  Males: n = 44 (40%)
  Females: n = 66 (60%)
	44 revisions (1 re-revision)
	69 revisions (3 bilateral, 1 re-revision)
		—

Mean age at primary surgery Mean age at revision surgery	49.9 y (14–71) 52.5 y (18–71)	—
Primary diagnosis: N = 111 Re-revision: 2 cup revisions	Osteoarthritis: n = 95 (85.8%) Congenital hip dysplasia: n = 7 (6.2%) Avascular necrosis: n = 8 (7.1%) Rheumatoid arthritis: n = 1 (0.9%) 1 cup loosening, 1 head loosening	—

Types of hip resurfacing: N =113	Overall number	KADS: N = 43	% of total number by KADS 43/3313 resurf = 1.3%
BHR	n = 61 (55.8%)	n = 31	31/1967 BHR = 1.6%
McMinn	n = 2 (1.8%)	—	—
Conserve® Plus	n = 19 (16.8%)	n = 8	8/1055 = 0.8%
Conserve® Plus A-Class®	n = 1 (0.9%)	n = 1	1/122 = 0.8%
ASR	n = 10 (8.8%)	n = 2	2/66 = 3.0%
DUROM	n = 10 (8.8%)	—	—
ADEPT	n = 4 (3.5%)	—	—
CORMET 2000	n = 3 (2.6%)	—	—
RECAP	n = 3 (2.6%)	n = 1	1/18 = 5.6%
—	2 re-revisions of BHR resurfacings		

Abbreviation: KADS, K.A. De Smet (primary surgeon).

months). The 2 cases of re-revision were conducted at 22 and 27 months after the first revision.

Diagnostic Tools

The diagnostic assessment of patients with a painful or failed hip resurfacing included plain anteroposterior and false-profile standing radiographs, clinical examination and scoring (Harris Hip Score [HHS][14]), and serum metal ion measurements (Chromium [Cr] and Cobalt [Co]) done routinely since 2005/2006. Metal ion measurements were performed at the Laboratory for Toxicology of the University of Ghent, Belgium. Levels higher than 5.1 μg/L for Cr and 4.4 μg/L for Co were considered to be elevated and possibly associated with clinical problems due to increased wear of the components (De Smet KA, Campbell PA, van Orsouw M, et al. Interpretation of metal ion levels after metal-on-metal resurfacing. Poster presentation at the America Academy for Orthopaedic Surgeons. New Orleans [LA], March 2010, unpublished data). The radiographs were analyzed for acetabular and femoral component positioning with inclination and anteversion angles, femoral neck fracture or progressive neck narrowing, component migration or subsidence, and radiolucent lines, osteolytic lesions, or signs of bone remodeling. To assess the position of the acetabular components accurately and objectively, an EBRA analysis (Einzel Bild Roentgen Analyze, University of Innsbruck, Innsbruck, Austria)[15,16] was performed by an independent reader (G.G.), who measured both the cup inclination and version angles. Optimal placement of the acetabular component was defined an inclination of 45° and an anteversion of 20°. A "safe zone" was defined as a zone of ± 10° about the optimum orientation. Components placed outside the safe zone were considered to be malpositioned.

When an infection or a soft tissue reaction was suspected, additional investigations were performed, including total body bone scans and granulocyte scans to investigate a possible infection, and ultrasonography and/or magnetic resonance imaging to look for cysts or soft tissue masses.

Retrieved periprosthetic tissues were sent to an independent laboratory for retrieval analysis,[17] histologic examination, and ALVAL (Aseptic Lymphocytic Vasculitis Associated Lesions) scoring.[18]

Surgical Procedures

During the revision operation, a posterolateral approach was used for 110 interventions and an anterolateral for 3 (**Table 2**). Whenever possible, it was attempted to preserve well-fixed, well-positioned acetabular and femoral components. When the acetabular component had to be revised, it was carefully removed with chisels to minimize loss of bone stock. Encapsulated fluid collections and metal-stained, damaged periprosthetic tissues were excised completely in the early revisions. With increasing experience, however, dissection was done with the utmost care to preserve as much muscle and soft tissue as possible to sustain the stability of the hip. Among the 113 hip resurfacing revisions, 10 (8.8%) were cup-only, 22 (19.5%) were femoral component-only revision, and the remaining 81 (71.7%) had both components revised. A ceramic-on-ceramic hybrid total hip replacement was used in 11 cases (9.7% of total revisions) with an uncemented acetabular component. Seventy-one uncemented total hip replacements were performed, 5 had Big Femoral Head metal-on-metal (MoM) bearings, and the remainder were ceramic-on-ceramic (CoC). The head diameters of the revision hips ranged from 28 to 58 mm with a mean diameter of 39.8 mm (median 36 mm).

Following the initial experience[13] there was a difference in surgical practice. There were significantly fewer cup-only revisions (7 vs 3) ($P<.001$), a greater number of uncemented, titanium, THA stems were implanted ($P<.001$), and bigger THA femoral heads were used ($P = .01$).

Postoperative Care

Postoperative rehabilitation and thromboprophylaxis were performed following a routine hip arthroplasty protocol. Patients with a revision to a total hip replacement in whom both the acetabular and femoral component had been revised with decrease of the femoral head size, and patients in whom the hip capsule and soft tissue had been removed due to extensive metallosis and tissue necrosis, were asked to wear an antidislocation hip abduction brace for 6 weeks. This measure was taken following 5 cases of dislocation after hip resurfacing revisions in the early series, of which the results have been reported.[13] All revised patients are reviewed clinically and radiographically at 6 weeks and subsequently at 1, 2, and 5 years postoperatively.

Outcome Measures

Patient-reported clinical outcome was assessed with the harris hip score (HHS).[14] HHS was obtained prior to revision and at clinical reviews. The change in HHS (ΔHHS) between preoperative and latest follow-up was defined as: ΔHHS = $HHS_{follow-up} - HHS_{pre-revision}$.

The mean follow up after revision was 43 months (range 3–121 months).

Data were collected prospectively for all cases. Complications and re-revisions were recorded.

Analyses

Outcome was compared for gender, revision type, and operative findings, more specifically the presence or absence of soft tissue fluid collections.

Analysis was also performed for different subgroups: the first 42 cases, previously reported,[13] comprised the Initial Group, the initial

---

Table 2
Revision procedures

Type of Revision Procedure	Number
Cup-only	n = 10 (8.8%)
Femoral stem with Big Femoral Head metal-on-metal	n = 22 (19.5%)
Total hip revision	n = 81 (including 2 re-revisions) (71.7%)
Hybrid THA (cemented stem) all ceramic-on-ceramic bearings	n = 11 (9.7%)
Uncemented THA	n = 70 (61.7%)
With Conserve® Plus Big Femoral Head metal-on-metal	n = 5
With ceramic-on-ceramic bearing	n = 65
Head diameters of revision components	Mean 39.8 mm (28–58)
28–36 mm ceramic head	n = 58 (51.3%)
38–58 mm ceramic or metal head	n = 55 (48.7%)

experience of revisions of failed hip resurfacings. Cases from 43 onwards formed the Later Group.

Patients with metal ion levels used as a diagnostic tool formed the Ions-measured Group (n = 74) and the outcome of these patients were compared with the outcome of patients without ion levels (Ions-not-measured Group, n = 36).

Nonparametric statistical tests were used to analyze HHS, femoral head size, time to revision, and so forth. The Chi-squared test was used for complication and re-revision rates. Significance was considered when P values of less than .05 were obtained; all statistical analyses were performed using SPSS (version 18, IBM SPSS, Chicago, IL, USA).

RESULTS
Reasons for Revision

One hundred and six patients (109 hips) presented with some degree of pain or discomfort in the hip region, often associated with mechanical symptoms such as impingement or limited range of motion, and in a few cases also with a swelling around the groin (**Table 3**). Four patients had no pain symptoms. The mean HHS before revision was 70.4 points (range 25–100). Elevated metal ion levels with or without radiographic signs of failure were an indication for revision in cases without clinical symptoms. Overall the metal ions levels were elevated in 40 patients (54.1%). The mean Cr levels were 22.39 µg/L (range 0.5–146.0 with a median of 7.40 µg/L) and the mean Co levels 22.42 µg/L (range 0.5–119.0 with a median of 4.40 µg/L). In the 40 patients with high metal ions, impingement was established intraoperatively in 11 cases (27.5%), metallosis in 36 cases (90%), and an adverse soft tissue reaction in 32 cases (80%).

The most common indication for revision was a symptomatic patient with a malpositioned cup (n = 68 cases, 60%). The most common radiological finding was osteolysis (n = 57, 50.4%), noted either as progressive neck narrowing, as radiolucent lines around the components, or as osteolytic lesions. Metal ions above the safe levels of 5.1 µg/L Cr or 4.4 µg/L Co (De Smet KA, Campbell PA, van Orsouw M, et al. Interpretation of metal ion levels after metal-on-metal resurfacing. Poster presentation at the America Academy for Orthopaedic Surgeons. New Orleans [LA], March 2010, unpublished data) were found in 40 patients (54.1% of all metal ion measurements). In 3 cases (2.6%) high metal ion levels were the primary reason for revision. Fifteen of the 48 soft tissue fluid collections (31.3%) were encountered with cups positioned in the safe zone. Six of those were found to be

Table 3 Reasons for revisions and intraoperative findings	
Preoperative Reason for Revision	**Number and Percentage**
More than 1 reason	n = 19 (16.5%)
Cup malpositioning	n = 57 (49.6%)
Cup loosening	n = 15 (13.0%)
Head malpositioning	n = 11 (9.6%)
Head loosening	n = 21 (18.3%)
Osteolysis	n = 57 (49.6%)
Fracture	n = 6 (5.2%)
Infection	n = 6 (5.2%)
Mismatch	n = 1 (0.9%)
High metal ions (measured since 2005–6)	n = 40 (34.8%)
Pain	n = 19 (16.5%)
Pain as only reason	n = 1 (0.9%)
Intra- and Postoperative Findings	**Number and Percentage**
Osteolysis	n = 33 (28.6%)
Neck narrowing	n = 20 (17.4%)
Impingement	n = 39 (33.9%)
Oversized components	n = 4 (3.5%)
Metallosis	n = 37 (30.8%)
Soft tissue fluid collection	n = 48 (42.5%)
Metal sensitivity	n = 6 (5.2%)

related to metal sensitivity (1 bilateral) and 3 to femoral component loosening; 6 others had high metal ions with or without signs of neck narrowing or impingement.

Surgical Observations

The most common intraoperative findings were a cystic soft tissue reaction (n = 48, 42.5%) and impingement (n = 37, 30.6%) (see **Table 3**). Cystic soft tissue fluid collections (**Fig. 2**) around the hip were seen with all designs. The 3 female patients with bilateral revisions had bilateral soft tissue reactions. Soft tissue collections were associated with less soft tissue destruction in the Later Group.

Time Intervals to Revision

The mean time interval between the primary hip resurfacing arthroplasty and the first revision was 30.9 months, ranging from 0 (1 case of mismatch) to 101 months (median 23 months) (**Table 4**). Femoral neck fractures occurred early postoperatively with a mean time to revision of 2.5 months

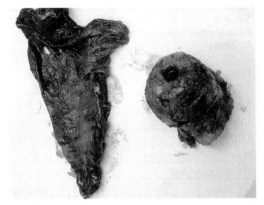

Fig. 2. Cystic soft tissue reaction (bursa) with pronounced metallosis from a patient with a malpositioned BHR revised at 56 months.

(range 1–9 months). The overall time to revision related to increased wear and/or reactions to metal debris (with exclusion of fractures, infections, and head loosening) was 32.5 months (range 4–101 months). When these soft tissue reactions were found with cups outside of the safe zone and with high metal ion levels, the time to revision was shorter (mean 40 months) than with soft tissue reactions with well-positioned cups (mean 67 months: $P = .037$).

In 88% of cases (n = 101) the problems leading to failure and revision of the hip resurfacing arthroplasty occurred within 5 years postoperatively. A case of ASR hip resurfacing revision is illustrated in **Figs. 3–5**.

Clinical Outcome and Complications

The HHS increased from a mean of 70.4 preoperatively to 93.1 postoperatively (HHS$_{follow-up}$; range 42–100, median 96 points) ($P<.001$) with a mean ΔHHS of 23.2 (**Tables 5** and **6**). A total of 11 complications (9.7%) occurred. Dislocation was the most common complication, occurring in 5

cases, all in CoC THA with heads 36 mm or smaller. Six re-revisions were performed. Both males and females had good outcome after revision surgery; there was no difference in HHS$_{follow-up}$ ($P = .78$), ΔHHS ($P = .14$), and complication or re-revision rates ($P = .63$).

There was no difference in HHS$_{follow-up}$ ($P = .78$), ΔHHS ($P = .64$), or complication rates ($P = .6$) between the different revision types (cup-only, stem-only, both components). However, there was a higher re-revision rate in single-component revisions in comparison with both-component revisions ($P = .045$). Outcome comparison between different bearing options demonstrated increased complication and re-revision rates when THA with a MoM large-diameter femoral head was used in cases other than fractures ($P = .035$).

For the whole cohort, the presence of a soft tissue fluid collection did not significantly affect outcome ($P = .65$).

Subgroup Analysis

Outcome was significantly better in the Later Group than in the Initial Group, as demonstrated by significantly better HHS$_{follow-up}$ ($P = .04$) (see **Table 5**). Of the 11 complications, 8 occurred in the Initial Group, of which 5 had to be re-revised. There was a significant reduction in complication and re-revision rates ($P = .01$) in the Later Group (see **Table 6**).

Amongst patients with soft-tissue fluid collections, the ones in the Later Group (n = 31) had significantly reduced complication ($P = .005$) and re-revision ($P = .016$) rates compared with the Initial Group (n = 17).

There was no difference in HHS ($P = .47$) and ΔHHS ($P = .45$) between the patients of the Ions-measured and the Ions-not-measured Groups. However, the incidence of complications and re-revisions was significantly reduced in the Ions-measured Group ($P = .004$).

DISCUSSION

This single-surgeon consecutive series of revisions of hip resurfacing arthroplasties aimed to determine outcome following revision for a variety of modes of failure and to identify factors that improve outcome post-revision.

Acetabular component malpositioning in symptomatic patients with soft tissue reactions was the leading cause for revision in the authors' specialist referral center. These reactions are now acknowledged as the principal reasons for midterm failure of hip resurfacing arthroplasties.[5,13,19] Cup malpositioning has been demonstrated to

Table 4 Time between index hip resurfacing operation and revision	
	Mean Time to Revision
Overall	30.9 mo (0–101)
Fractures	2.5 mo (1–9)
For reasons of malpositioning or wear (fracture, infection, head loosening excluded)	Overall 32.5 mo (4–101)

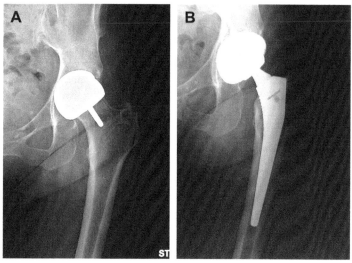

Fig. 3. Radiographs of an ASR hip resurfacing in a 49-year-old female patient with osteoarthritis. Cup malpositioning with excessive inclination and anteversion and high metal ion levels Cr 56.9 μg/L and Co 72.4 μg/L. Revision to a ceramic bearing noncemented THA was performed at 22 months. (*A*) Pre-revision radiograph: inclination of 58° and anteversion of 23° (EBRA). (*B*) Post-revision radiograph: inclination of 49° and anteversion of 27° (EBRA).

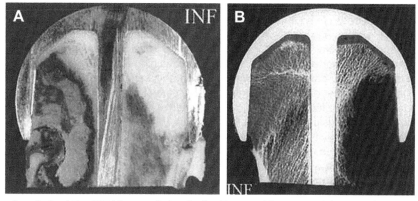

Fig. 4. Retrieval analysis of the ASR hip resurfacing in the 49-year-old woman with cup malpositioning revised at 22 months. Photograph (*A*) and radiograph (*B*) of a cross section through the retrieved femoral head showing osteolysis and invasion by soft tissue. (*Courtesy of* Pat Campbell, PhD, Los Angeles, CA.)

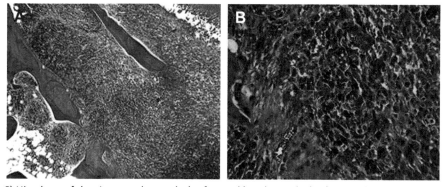

Fig. 5. (*A, B*) Histology of the tissue underneath the femoral head reveals the femoral head is viable and vascular, but the bone is being resorbed by invasive metal-filled macrophages (ALVAL) (*A*, hematoxylin-eosin, original magnification ×40; *B*, hematoxylin-eosin, original magnification ×200). (*Courtesy of* Pat Campbell, PhD, Los Angeles, CA.)

Table 5
Clinical outcome

	HHS Pre-Revision	HHS Follow-Up	ΔHHS
All hips (N = 113)	Mean 70.4 (25–100)	Mean 93.1 (42–100)	23.2 (−31[a]–75)
Initial Group (n = 42)	Mean 72.6 (40–96)	Mean 90.7 (42–100)	18.1 (−31[a]–56)
Later Group (n = 71)	Mean 68.8 (25–100)	Mean 94.7 (64–100)[b]	26.0 (0–75)

[a] Case of post-revision infection that was reoperated.
[b] Significantly better in Later Group than Initial Group (P = .04).

lead to higher wear of the articulatingsurfaces due to edge loading,[5,20] generating metal particles and higher levels of circulating metal ions. As a reaction to this metal debris, soft tissue reactions, either cystic or solid, metallosis of the periprosthetic tissues, and osteolysis may occur. In this series soft tissue reactions, definitely related to enhanced wear and metal debris, were found around 48 hips in 45 patients. Most of those reactions were seen with malpositioned cups but 15 (31.3%) were found with well-oriented components, related either to metal sensitivity, femoral component loosening, or high metal ion levels with or without signs of neck narrowing or impingement. Similar observations have been reported before[21,22] with masses in well-positioned components, which have led to the search for additional tribological and biomechanical causative factors.[5,6,20]

Metal debris may illicit sensitivity reactions, but these are rare. Metal sensitivity as a reason for hip resurfacing revision was established in 5 patients in this series (one with bilateral soft tissue reaction); all were females who had low ion levels, cystic collections, and high ALVAL score.

Although femoral neck fractures are the most frequent cause for early revision,[23] the small number of fractures in this series (**Table 7**) reflects the small incidence of fracture by the senior surgeon (n = 3, incidence: 0.1%).

High metal ions levels were seen in 54% of patients tested (n = 74). There was a strong correlation between presence of soft tissue fluid collection and high ions (r = 0.64, P<.001). The presence of high ions in a symptomatic hip had a fourfold risk of having a collection. These findings confirm the importance of metal ion measurements in the assessment of hip resurfacings and in predicting a soft tissue reaction before it becomes symptomatic. Metal ions can hence aid surgeons, along with other investigations, to decide whether and when to revise an HRA to prevent extensive soft tissue damage. A clinical algorithm has been designed to assist surgeons when reviewing a problematic hip resurfacing (**Fig. 6**).

In this series, soft tissue collections found with high metal ion levels had a shorter time to revision when associated with malpositioned cups than with well-positioned cups (P = .037). This finding confirms the fact that combination of a radiographic diagnosis of cup malpositioning with elevated metal ion levels is a valuable reason to revise an HRA at an earlier stage, thereby preventing extensive soft tissue destruction to occur.

In general, the outcome of the hip resurfacing revisions was very good, with a significant improvement of the HHS compared with the preoperative values (mean 93, range 42–100) (P<.001). The complication rate was 10% and the re-revision rate was 5% at a mean follow-up of 43 months.

Table 6
Complications and re-revisions

Complications (N = 11)	Initial Group	Re-Revised	Later Group	Re-Revised
Dislocation	4 (1 twice)	1	1	–
Component loosening	2	2	–	–
Infection	1	1	2	1
Metal sensitivity	1	1		
Re-revisions n = 6		5		1

Table 7
Comparison of Australian Joint Replacement Registry 2010 annual report and ANCA clinic series (Dr Koen De Smet)

Reason for Revision	Australian Joint Register 2010		ANCA Clinic, Ghent, Belgium	
	N	%	N	%
Fracture	195	35.6	6	5.3
Loosening/Lysis	183	33.4	31[a]	27.4
Infection	45	8.2	6	5.3
Metal sensitivity	39	7.1	6	5.3
Pain	29	5.3	4	3.5
Avascular necrosis	17	3.1	[b]	[b]
Prosthesis dislocation	15	2.7	1	0.9
Malposition	12	2.2	54	47.9
Other	13	1.1	5[c]	4.4
Total	548	100.0	113 revisions	100.0

[a] Loosening/lysis cases minus the 6 cases of metal allergy.
[b] Avascular necrosis of head is counted in Loosening/Lysis.
[c] Other (1 mismatch and 4 high metal ion levels) as most important reason for revision.

There was no difference in outcome between genders. Although data from registries[1,2,12] and individual series,[7,8,19] including the current one, have shown increased failure rates amongst females, the results of this study show that both genders have good outcome following revision, with similarly low complication rates.

De Steiger and colleagues[12] demonstrated a difference in survival between different types of revisions, and this study supports part of their findings. Single-part revisions (cup-only and femoral component-only) have an increased re-revision risk, and careful patient and indication selections should be applied when surgeons decide for single-component revisions, especially in cases other than early fracture. Forty-three revisions had their primaries by the senior surgeon, allowing for full chronologic history in these cases. Amongst those, there was a greater proportion of females (73%, $P = .03$), and a greater number of acetabular components was within the previously described safe-zone in comparison with those referred from elsewhere ($P = .001$). However, there were no differences in intraoperative findings or clinical outcome between this group and the patients referred from elsewhere.

Five dislocations occurred early in the series (Initial Group). Analysis of these cases led to the conclusion that the dislocations were related to the reduction of the hip stability for several reasons. The hip resurfacings had been revised to CoC THAs with a femoral head size of 28 to 36 mm. Ceramic implants were preferred to large-diameter MoM heads in these patients, to avoid a further burden of metal particles and ions. Moreover, because metallosis had invaded the periprosthetic tissues including the hip capsule, the affected tissues were removed during the revision procedure, thereby decreasing the stability of the hip joint.

In other series especially reporting on patients with extensive soft tissue reactions,[4] worse clinical outcomes with high complication (25%) and re-revision rates (21%) were described. The findings of this series confirm that the outcome of revisions in cases with extensive tissue destruction during the surgeon's learning curve (Initial Group) had significantly increased complication (19%) and re-revision (12%) rates. However, greater experience (Later Group), translating to the use of a clinical evaluation algorithm, revision at an earlier stage, bigger THA ceramic heads, and patient education, improved the complication (4.2%) and re-revision rate (1.4%).

As the total number of primary resurfacing procedures is increasing globally, the number of revisions is bound to increase, as shown this study. Failure rates vary with different experience levels, with low-volume surgeons having greater failure rates.[1,24] This study, showing a learning curve to outcome following revision, would support an argument in favor of revisions of failing hip resurfacings to be performed only by centers experienced with such complications in order to improve outcome.

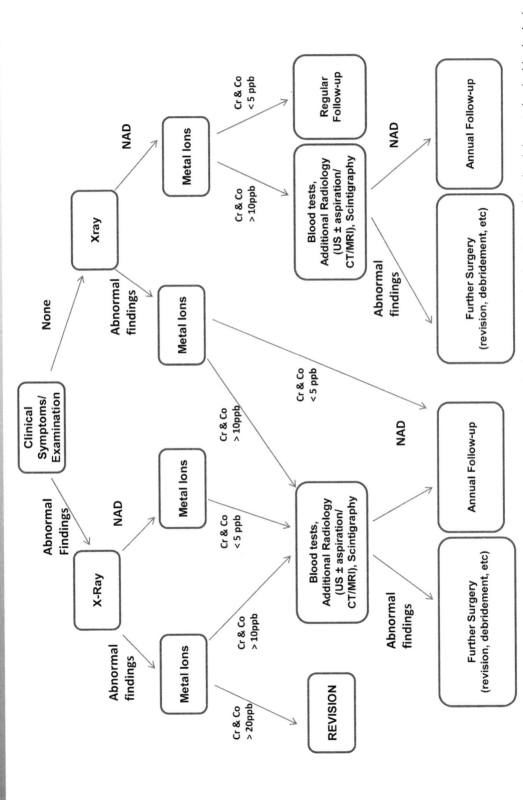

Fig. 6. Clinical algorithm for the review a problematic hip resurfacing. Before making the decision to revise the HRA, metal ion levels have to be double-checked and correctly interpreted with exclusion of other sources including other CoCr implants and elevated levels secondary to renal impairment. NAD, no abnormalities diagnosed. NAD, no abnormalities diagnosed.

SUMMARY

Malpositioning of components with associated wear-induced soft tissue fluid collections was the most frequent factor leading to failure of a hip resurfacing arthroplasty. Mid-term outcome following revision is good, and complication and re-revision rates can be low. Surgical experience, early intervention in cases of malpositioned implants, clinical use of ion levels, implantation of larger CoC THA femoral heads, and patient education are factors in improving outcome and reducing complication and re-revisions following HRA revision.

ACKNOWLEDGMENTS

The authors express their special thanks to Dr Pat Campbell (Implant Retrieval Center, Los Angeles, CA, USA) for the analysis of the retrieved components and the histologic analyses.

REFERENCES

1. Australian Orthopaedic Association National Joint Replacement Registry. Annual report. 2010. Available at: http://www.aoa.org.au. Accessed January 5, 2011.
2. National Joint Registry for England and Wales. 7th annual report. 2010. Available at: http://www.njrcentre.org.uk. Accessed January 5, 2011.
3. Ollivere B, Darrah C, Barker T, et al. Early clinical failure of the Birmingham metal-on-metal hip resurfacing is associated with metallosis and soft-tissue necrosis. J Bone Joint Surg Br 2009;91:1025–30.
4. Grammatopoulos G, Pandit H, Kwon Y-M, et al. Hip resurfacings revised for inflammatory pseudotumour have a poor outcome. J Bone Joint Surg Br 2009;91:1019–24.
5. De Haan R, Pattyn C, Gill HS, et al. Correlation between inclination of the acetabular component and metal ion levels in metal-on-metal hip resurfacing replacement. J Bone Joint Surg Br 2009;91:1287–95.
6. Griffin WL, Nanson CJ, Springer BD, et al. Reduced articular surface of one-piece cups. A cause of runaway wear and early failure. Clin Orthop Relat Res 2010;468(9):2328–32.
7. McBryde CW, Theivendran K, Thomas AMC, et al. The influence of head size and sex on the outcome of Birmingham hip resurfacing. J Bone Joint Surg Am 2010;92:105–12.
8. Jameson SS, Langton D, Natu S, et al. The Influence of age and sex on early clinical results after hip resurfacing. An independent center analysis. J Arthroplasty 2008;23(6 Suppl 1):50–5.
9. Daniel J, Ziaee H, Pradhan C, et al. Blood and urine metal ion levels in young and active patients after Birmingham hip resurfacing arthroplasty. Four-year results of a prospective longitudinal study. J Bone Joint Surg Br 2007;89:169–73.
10. De Smet K, de Haan R, Calistri A, et al. Metal ion measurement as a diagnostic tool to identify problems with metal-on-metal hip resurfacing. J Bone Joint Surg Am 2008;90:202–8.
11. Ball ST, Le Duff MJ, Amstutz HC. Early results of conversion of a failed femoral component in hip resurfacing arthroplasty. J Bone Joint Surg Am 2007; 89:735–41.
12. de Steiger RN, Miller LN, Prosser GH, et al. Poor outcome of revised resurfacing hip arthroplasty. 397 cases from the Australian Joint Replacement Registry. Acta Orthop 2010;81(1):72–6.
13. de Haan R, Campbell PA, Su EP, et al. Revision of metal-on-metal resurfacing arthroplasty of the hip. J Bone Joint Surg Br 2008;90:1158–63.
14. Harris WH. Traumatic arthritis of the hip after dislocation and acetabular fractures: treatment by mold arthroplasty. An end-result study using a new method of result evaluation. J Bone Joint Surg Am 1969;51: 737–55.
15. Krismer M, Bauer R, Tschupik J, et al. EBRA: a method to measure migration of acetabular components. J Biomech 1995;28:1225–72.
16. Biedermann R, Krismer M, Stockl B, et al. Accuracy of EBRA-FCA in the measurement of migration of femoral components of total hip replacement. Einzel-Bild-Röntgen-Analyse-femoral component analysis. J Bone Joint Surg Br 1999;81:266–72.
17. Campbell PA, Beaulé PE, Ebramzadeh E. A study of implant failure in metal-on-metal surface arthroplasties. Clin Orthop 2006;453:35–46.
18. Campbell PA, Ebramzadeh E, Nelson S, et al. Histological features of pseudotumor-like tissues from metal-on-metal hips. Clin Orthop Relat Res 2010; 468(9):2321–7.
19. Carrothers AD, Gilbert RE, Jaiswal A, et al. Birmingham hip resurfacing. The prevalence of failure. J Bone Joint Surg Br 2010;92:1344–50.
20. Langton DJ, Sprowson AP, Joyce TJ, et al. Blood metal in concentrations after hip resurfacing arthroplasty: a comparative study of articular surface replacement and Birmingham Hip Resurfacing arthroplasties. J Bone Joint Surg Br 2009;91:1287–95.
21. Pandit H, Glynn-Jones S, McLardy-Smith P, et al. Pseudotumours associated with metal-on-metal hip resurfacings. J Bone Joint Surg Br 2008;90(7):847–51.
22. Grammatopoulos G, Pandit H, Glynn-Jones S, et al. Optimal acetabular orientation for hip resurfacing. J Bone Joint Surg Br 2010;92(8):1072–8.
23. Steffen RT, Foguet PR, Krikler SJ, et al. Femoral neck fractures after hip resurfacing. J Arthroplasty 2009; 24(4):614–9.
24. Shimmin AJ, Graves S, Noble PC. The effect of operative volume on the outcome of hip resurfacing. J Arthroplasty 2010;25(3):e4.

The Future of Hip Resurfacing

Thomas P. Schmalzried, MD[a,b,*]

KEYWORDS

- Hip resurfacing • Metal-metal bearing • Wear
- Component positioning

During the first 10 years of experience with metal-metal hip resurfacing, several important observations were made that influence the future of hip resurfacing.[1] Patient characteristics significantly affected survival. Patients younger than 65 years and those of larger stature, most commonly men with osteoarthritis, have had the best prognosis. Smaller stature and small component size have been associated with a higher risk of short-term failure. Surgical experience with resurfacing significantly improves patient outcomes, mostly by the elimination of short-term complications such as femoral neck fracture, dislocation, and loosening. Cobalt-chromium alloy monoblock acetabular components are more challenging to insert properly than modular titanium alloy components. A resurfacing acetabular component that is less than 5 mm thick requires bone removal (reaming) equivalent to total hip replacement. Component position (femoral-acetabular mating) and design influences the bearing wear, ion level, and occurrence of an adverse local tissue reaction (ALTR).[2]

academic programs. Education for metal-metal resurfacing was primarily through industry-sponsored courses, with a variable degree of supervised surgery on actual patients. All orthopedic residents receive training in total hip replacement, but training in hip resurfacing is not available to many. Residency training should include the fundamentals of patient selection for resurfacing, preoperative planning, and avoidance and management of complications. The greatest benefit of residency training, however, is in the operating room. The best way to learn surgical skills is through direct observation and repetition of the correct technique under the guidance of an experienced mentor. This deficit in residency training should be considered when comparing community results (ie, joint registries) of total hip replacement with hip resurfacing. Regardless of technological evolution, the outcomes of community hip resurfacings would be improved if the steep portion of the learning curve occurs during residency training.

EDUCATION AND REDUCING THE LEARNING CURVE

There is a need for better education on hip resurfacing in residency training programs. The learning curve for most surgical procedures occurs during residency. When metal-metal resurfacing became available, a paucity of practicing orthopedic surgeons had prior training in hip resurfacing.[3] There are limitations on surgical training outside

SURGICAL TECHNIQUE, COMPONENT POSITIONING, AND INSTRUMENTATION

Most short-term complications associated with resurfacing, including femoral neck fractures, dislocation, loosening, accelerated wear, and ALTRs, are related to surgical technique or component position.[2] On the femoral side, varus component orientation, neck notching, overpenetration of cement, and vigorous femoral impaction should

---

[a] Joint Replacement Institute at St Vincent Medical Center, 2200 West Third Street, Suite 400, Los Angeles, CA 90057, USA
[b] Department of Orthopaedic Surgery, Harbor-UCLA Medical Center, 1000 West Carson Street, Box 422, Torrance, CA 90509, USA
* Corresponding author. Joint Replacement Institute at St Vincent Medical Center, 2200 West Third Street, Suite 400, Los Angeles, CA 90057.
E-mail address: schmalzried@earthlink.net

Orthop Clin N Am 42 (2011) 271–273
doi:10.1016/j.ocl.2010.12.004

be avoided.[4-8] The currently available mechanical means for femoral guide pin placement have a learning curve.[9] Computer-assisted (navigation) femoral guide pin placement improves accuracy when compared with mechanical means.[10] Preoperative 3-dimensional analysis of the proximal femur using computed tomography or magnetic resonance imaging creates a shape-matching guide for femoral pin placement.[11] This methodology is more time efficient than intraoperative computer navigation.

The prime problem in hip arthroplasty today is acetabular component positioning.[12] Because of the relatively small head to neck ratio of resurfacing compared with modern total hip replacement, the window for proper component position is smaller. There are 2 challenges: determining the desired component positions for a specific hip and being able to reliably implant the components in that position. Current evidence indicates that the determination of satisfactory femoral-acetabular mating includes consideration of the native femoral valgus and the corresponding acetabular component lateral opening and the native femoral version and the corresponding acetabular component version. To achieve adequate bearing contact area, a femur with increased valgus needs a correspondingly lower acetabular component lateral opening angle. Similarly, a femur with increased anteversion needs a correspondingly lower acetabular component anteversion.[13]

Inserting the acetabular component into the desired position requires identification of the pelvic plane or the use of validated surrogates. Innovations to accomplish this positioning include mechanical guides,[14] intraoperative imaging,[1] computer-assisted surgery (navigation),[13] and pelvic/acetabular shape-matching guides.

Monoblock acetabular components with a cobalt-chromium alloy substrate are more difficult to properly seat than modular titanium alloy total hip replacement components. This disparity is because of the increased stiffness of the cobalt chrome components, the absence of a dome hole to visually assess the seating, and the relatively bulky monoblock insertion devices, which limit peripheral visualization and impinge on adjacent tissues. Future innovations include alternative means to assess seating and debulking with easily reattachable insertion/extraction instrumentation.

CEMENTLESS FEMORAL FIXATION

Although several centers report high survival at more than 10 years with a cemented femoral component,[15] interest remains in cementless femoral fixation. A cementless femoral component avoids the reported inconsistencies and complications associated with cementing. Multisurgeon experience is needed to demonstrate the relative benefits and risks of cementless femoral resurfacing.

BEARING SURFACES

The variable exposure to metal particles and ions associated with metal-metal resurfacing components continues to be a concern. A challenge for hip resurfacing is keeping an aggregate acetabular component thickness of 5 mm or less (acetabular-femoral component outer to inner diameter difference of ≤10 mm) to conserve acetabular bone stock. There is limited experience with ceramic-ceramic hip resurfacing. The enthusiasm for the low wear potential and biocompatibility of these materials is tempered by fracture risk in the young and active, predominantly male (larger stature), patient undergoing resurfacing. Ceramic-on-metal bearings for total hip replacement (metallic acetabular component) demonstrate very low wear in simulator tests.[16,17] This bearing couple can be extended to hip resurfacing. Clinical data are needed to assess the wear, ion production, position sensitivity, and survival compared with metal-metal and ceramic-ceramic implant systems. Oxinium-on-Oxinium implant (oxidized zirconium; Smith & Nephew, Memphis, TN, USA) has a potential application as a hip resurfacing bearing, with an acetabular component thickness of less than 5 mm.

There is now more than 10 years of clinical experience with cross-linked polyethylenes documenting low wear and reduced osteolysis.[18] The industry has slowly moved to the use of thinner modular liners to accommodate larger femoral heads. The clinical results with bearings of thickness 36 mm or more have been favorable to date. Wear simulator data indicate lower wear with thinner cross-linked polyethylene.[19] The minimum bearing thickness continues to be debated and is a function of the supporting substrate as well as the polyethylene material. A cementless monoblock acetabular component with a cross-linked polyethylene bearing and a thickness of less than 5 mm would be attractive for resurfacing. The femoral bearing could be a low-wear ceramic material. Such an embodiment would be particularly attractive in smaller sizes and in women, who have a higher risk of an ALTR with metal-metal resurfacing.[20]

REFERENCES

1. Mont MA, Schmalzried TP. Modern metal-on-metal hip resurfacing: important observations from the first ten years. J Bone Joint Surg 2008;90(Suppl 3):3–11.

2. Schmalzried TP. Metal-metal bearing surfaces in hip arthroplasty. Orthopedics 2009;32(9). Available at: http://www.orthosupersite.com/view.asp?rID=42831. Accessed December 21, 2010.

3. Della Valle CJ, Nunley RM, Raterman SJ, et al. Initial American experience with hip resurfacing following FDA approval [erratum in: Clin Orthop Relat Res 2009;467(2):587]. Clin Orthop Relat Res 2009; 467(1):72–8.

4. Amstutz HC, Campbell PA, Le Duff MJ. Fracture of the neck of the femur after surface arthroplasty of the hip. J Bone Joint Surg Am 2004;86(9): 1874–7.

5. Beaulé PE, Lee JL, Le Duff MJ, et al. Orientation of the femoral component in surface arthroplasty of the hip. A biomechanical and clinical analysis. J Bone Joint Surg Am 2004;86(9):2015–21.

6. Morlock MM, Bishop N, Zustin J, et al. Modes of implant failure after hip resurfacing: morphological and wear analysis of 267 retrieval specimens. J Bone Joint Surg Am 2008;90(Suppl 3):89–95.

7. Langton DJ, Jameson SS, Joyce TJ, et al. The effect of component size and orientation on the concentrations of metal ions after resurfacing arthroplasty of the hip. J Bone Joint Surg Br 2008; 90(9):1143–51.

8. Bitsch RG, Loidolt T, Heisel C, et al. Cementing techniques for hip resurfacing arthroplasty: in vitro study of pressure and temperature hip resurfacing: pressure and temperature. J Arthroplasty 2011;26(1):144–51.

9. Nunley RM, Zhu J, Brooks PJ, et al. The learning curve for adopting hip resurfacing among hip specialists. Clin Orthop Relat Res 2010;468(2): 382–91.

10. Olsen M, Chiu M, Gamble P, et al. A comparison of conventional guidewire alignment jigs with image-less computer navigation in hip resurfacing arthroplasty. J Bone Joint Surg Am 2010;92(9):1834–41.

11. Kunz M, Rudan JF, Xenoyannis GL, et al. Computer-assisted hip resurfacing using individualized drill templates. J Arthroplasty 2010;25(4):600–6.

12. Schmalzried TP. The importance of proper acetabular component positioning and the challenges to achieving it. Oper Tech Orthop 2009;19:132–6.

13. Dorr LD, Malik A, Dastane M, et al. Combined anteversion technique for total hip arthroplasty. Clin Orthop Relat Res 2009;467:119–27.

14. Steppacher SD, Kowal JH, Murphy SB. Improving cup positioning using a mechanical navigation instrument. Clin Orthop Relat Res 2011;469(2): 423–8.

15. Amstutz HC, Le Duff MJ, Campbell PA, et al. Clinical and radiographic results of metal-on-metal hip resurfacing with a minimum ten-year follow-up. J Bone Joint Surg Am 2010;92(16):2663–71.

16. Williams S, Schepers A, Isaac G, et al. The 2007 Otto Aufranc Award. Ceramic-on-metal hip arthroplasties: a comparative in vitro and in vivo study. Clin Orthop Relat Res 2007;465:23–32.

17. Isaac GH, Brockett C, Breckon A, et al. Ceramic-on-metal bearings in total hip replacement: whole blood metal ion levels and analysis of retrieved components. J Bone Joint Surg Br 2009;91(9):1134–41.

18. Bitsch RG, Loidolt T, Heisel C, et al. Reduction of osteolysis with use of Marathon cross-linked polyethylene. A concise follow-up, at a minimum of five years, of a previous report. J Bone Joint Surg Am 2008;90(7):1487–91.

19. Shen FW, Lu Z, McKellop HA. Wear versus thickness and other features of 5-Mrad crosslinked UHMWPE acetabular liners. Clin Orthop Relat Res 2011; 469(2):395–404.

20. Glyn-Jones S, Pandit H, Kwon YM, et al. Risk factors for inflammatory pseudotumour formation following hip resurfacing. J Bone Joint Surg Br 2009;91(12): 1566–74.

Index

orthopedic.theclinics.com

Orthop Clin N Am 42 (2011) 275–277
doi:10.1016/S0030-5898(11)00017-4
0030-5898/11/$ – see front matter © 2011 Elsevier Inc. All rights reserved.

Moving?

Make sure your subscription moves with you!

To notify us of your new address, find your **Clinics Account Number** (located on your mailing label above your name), and contact customer service at:

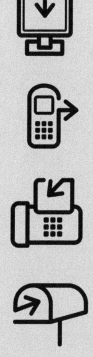

Email: journalscustomerservice-usa@elsevier.com

800-654-2452 (subscribers in the U.S. & Canada)
314-447-8871 (subscribers outside of the U.S. & Canada)

Fax number: 314-447-8029

Elsevier Health Sciences Division
Subscription Customer Service
3251 Riverport Lane
Maryland Heights, MO 63043

Printed and bound by CPI Group (UK) Ltd, Croydon, CR0 4YY

03/10/2024

01040357-0010